Quantum-Touch
The Power to Heal

By Richard Gordon

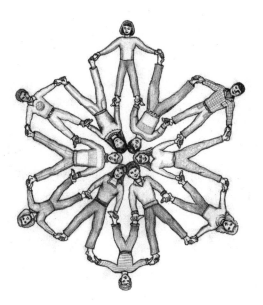

Illustrations by Eleanor Barrow
Cover by Eleanor Barrow and Carrie Toder

North Atlantic Books
Berkeley, California

In Praise of Quantum-Touch

"For professionals and lay people alike, Quantum-Touch is an essential and invaluable tool."

– Alternative Medicine Magazine, 2001

"Quantum-Touch is easy to learn, has a significant impact on the body's energy system and can make profound shifts in people's lives."

– Dr. Leonard Laskow, M.D.

"Every time I apply Quantum-Touch, I am in awe of the results. It's amazing how quickly the pain in my patients is resolved in just a few minutes."

– Roberta Horoho,
FNP, Physician Assistant

"In energy healing, the healer functions as a focusing lens for bioenergy, drawing such energy in and focusing that energy into the energy field of the person seeking healing. It is important for that lens to be as clear as possible. In its simplicity, Quantum-Touch slips past the healer's ego. This has the effect of increasing the clarity of the healer as a focusing lens. This effect makes Quantum-Touch a useful adjunct to other energy healing techniques as well as an excellent healing technique by itself. In its elegance, Quantum-Touch provides healing bioenergy for the healer as well as for the person seeking healing. Quantum-Touch could well be the current state-of-the-art technique in energy healing."

– Dr. Jerry Pittman, M.D.

"Quantum-Touch is an easily learnable skill that can provide balance, healing, comfort, and postural realignment. I salute Richard Gordon's unique gift for making difficult concepts readily accessible, and for his commitment to bringing this work to the world."

– David Kamnitzer, D.C.

"As an attorney, my training has led to a natural skepticism regarding so-called self-professed healers. After learning to do Quantum-Touch, however, I discovered a technique for directing healing energy that not only works, but which can be learned by anyone. I have been able to relieve my brother's chronic back pain. My girlfriend's heart palpitations and allergies have also responded well to this energy work. I highly recommend this to anyone."

– John W. Noretto, Esq.

"Quantum-Touch is an amazing method of healing – amazing because it's so simple to learn. You already possess the tools necessary to practice it and it works!"

– Sandra Alstrand, L.Ac.

"I love Quantum-Touch. I have dealt with energy medicine for many years since first studying polarity therapy, and Quantum-Touch is an exaltation of energy work. I use Quantum-Touch with my patients and family with excellent results."
– Habib Abdullah, D.C.

"Richard Gordon throws open the doors of energy healing for everyone. Simple techniques, profound results. Quantum-Touch is a system that anyone can learn quickly and put to use in their own lives."

– Chris Duffield, Ph.D.
Visiting Scholar, Stanford University

"Quantum-Touch accesses energy at a core level to promote surprisingly quick and effective healing. I highly recommend this method."

– Jacquelyn Lorell, L.Ac.

"Quantum-Touch makes a wonderfully powerful system readily and easily available to all. This book is a gift of illumination."

– Gloria Alvino, MS, R.Ph.

"In my vast experience, I've never seen anything to compare with the positive results of Quantum-Touch. It enabled affected team members to resume competitive play in a very brief period of time following an injury, and the improvements seemed to continue even after the therapeutic sessions."

– Duane Garner, Coach
UCSC Men's Basketball Team

"Richard Gordon has an unsurpassed ability for explaining energy healing to novices and professionals alike. Richard's first book, Your Healing Hands - The Polarity Experience, showed many of us how to use healing energy in our daily lives. Now Richard takes us on an even deeper journey, showing us how to activate the most profound levels of healing. He masterfully weaves together the story of his discoveries of Quantum-Touch with exceptionally clear illustrations that make it easy for anyone to learn this inspiring new technique. This book is invaluable to all health professionals. For the researcher, the phenomenon of Quantum-Touch represents an opportunity far too important to pass up."

– Jim Oschman, Ph.D.

"For energy medicine practitioners, Quantum-Touch amplifies the effects of Reiki and other hands-on healing techniques. For the layman, Quantum-Touch empowers the individual to tap into the innate healing abilities we all possess."

– Ellen DiNucci, M.A.
Project Coordinator, Complementary
and Alternative Medicine Program,
Stanford University

"Quantum-Touch is amazing! In just two days it successfully unfroze my shoulder which had not responded to several months of physical therapy and other healing modalities. It has now become an integral part of my practice and I would strongly recommend that everyone learn this easy and powerful technique."

– Billie Wolf, Occupational Therapist

"Quantum -Touch quickly and easily enables ordinary people to powerfully focus and amplify the life-force energy to become extraordinarily effective hands-on healers. For those who practice polarity therapy, massage, or therapeutic touch, your work can take on an astounding new dimension."

– Heather Wolfe, R.N., Lic. MT
Registered Polarity Therapy Instructor
Therapeutic Touch Instructor

"Far better than chiropractic, physical therapy, or medication, Quantum-Touch has completely relieved my chronic back pain. Quantum-Touch is a valuable asset to nurses who want to take a step forward in their careers and work on a much higher level. This should be studied in every nursing school across the country. Quantum-Touch is what is needed to transform the limited way nursing is currently practiced."

– Lauralyn C. McCurry
RNC, PHN, CARN

"When I combine Quantum-Touch with Reiki or cranial sacral therapy, my results are far more effective. Quantum-Touch awakens the magic in your hands."

– Roni Frank
Cranial Sacral Therapist,
Reiki Master

Dedication

I dedicate this book to the universal awareness that healing is not only real, but the easiest of skills to learn. With the awareness that the life-force is undeniable and tangible, I offer this book in support of the creation and establishment of a new branch of science based on the study of life-force energy: "Life-Force Science."

I believe that someday Life-Force Science will bring the dimension of consciousness to our understanding of physics, chemistry, biology, medicine, and psychology.

I gratefully dedicate this book to our shared future.

— *Richard Gordon*

Copyright

Quantum-Touch: The Power to Heal-Revised Edition
Copyright ©2002 by Richard Gordon

North Atlantic Books
P.O. Box 12327
Berkeley, California 94712

Disclaimer

This book is not intended to be a substitute for the services of health care professionals. Neither the author nor publisher is responsible for any consequences incurred by those employing the remedies or treatments reported herein. Any application of the material set forth in the following pages is at the reader's discretion and is his or her sole responsibility.

Quantum-Touch: The Power to Heal is distributed by the Society for the Study of Native Arts and Sciences, a non-profit educational corporation whose goals are to develop an educational and crosscultural perspecitve linking various scientific, social and artistic fields: to nurture a holistic view of arts, sciences, humanities, and healing; and to publish and distribute literature on the relationship of mind, body and nature.

Manufactured in the United States of America.

Library of Congress Cataloging in Publication Information

Gordon, Richard, 1948-
Quantum touch: the power to heal / Richard Gordon.
     p.   cm
ISBN 1-55643-393-x (alk. paper)
1. Imposition of hands--Therapeutic use. 2. Force and energy.
3. Healing. I. Title.
RZ999.G66   2002
615.8'9--dc21   99-30631
     CIP
3 4 5 6 7 / 02

Acknowlegments

Special thanks to Carrie Toder for book design, 11th hour layout angel, Sun McNamee. For editing, Elayne Crow, Laurel McCurrey, Betsy Aaron, and Kent Shew.

Contents

Foreword

Two decades ago, Delores Kreiger introduced the concept of Therapeutic Touch, which has been most widely used by nurses. Just as there are many roads to Rome, there are certainly many techniques for "healing." To me, all of these are part of a universal concept that I call "sacred healing."

I have personally met and have been trained by Richard Gordon in his healing modality, Quantum-Touch. Many of my staff also were trained and we were able to demonstrate that Quantum-Touch, even without touching the patient (!), is capable of changing the electroencephalogram. Symptomatic relief was obtained in a number of our chronic pain patients. Rapid relief of pain and resolution of healing after surgical removal of wisdom teeth was noted in one young lady. Sally Hammond in her book, We are All Healers, over 25 years ago emphasized the potential healing ability of every human being. Quantum-Touch appears to be the first technique that may truly allow us all to become healers.

Sincerely,
Dr. C. Norman Shealy, M.D., Ph.D.
Founder, Shealy Institute for Comprehensive Health Care
Founding President, American Holistic Medical Association
Research & Clinical Professor of Psychology,
Forest Institute of Professional Psychology

Introduction

Quantum-Touch is a method of hands-on healing that literally must be seen to be believed. Employing only a very light touch on yourself or others, you can profoundly accelerate the body's own healing response. The effect is so immediate and extraordinary, you can actually see bones in the body spontaneously realigning themselves with only a light touch. Since the body decides where to place these bones, you need never worry about doing it right. Beyond structural realignment, pain and inflammation are quickly reduced, while organs, systems, and glands become balanced.

To empower yourself to use Quantum-Touch, you simply need to learn various breathing techniques, body awareness meditations, and hand positions. Those who apply the principles and techniques of this book can become highly capable practitioners in but a single day. This is because the ability to heal is an inherent part of people's essential nature. Just as new cars coming off the assembly line are all equipped with a steering wheel, windows, and doors, the ability to help heal each other is automatically built into the system. As surely as children are endowed with the ability to walk, learn language, laugh, cry, and love, we all have the ability to be healing practitioners.

Once you have learned Quantum-Touch, you can never forget how to do it. The process is very much like learning to ride a bicycle. Before you begin, the idea of sitting upright on two skinny wheels would probably seem quite impossible. When you first start to stay upright, it seems like a miracle, but after some time, it becomes completely natural and expected. When you first observe the results of using Quantum-Touch, the experience will often be surprising and unforgettable. Like riding a bicycle, what had appeared miraculous will in time become natural and even expected. Beyond this, there is an immense joy and satisfaction in knowing that you can assist others in their healing process. One small note of caution: I believe that this joy is contagious.

Deepak Chopra wrote, *"To promote the healing response, you must get past all the grosser levels of the body — cells, tissues, organs, and systems — and arrive at a junction between mind and matter, the point where consciousness actually starts to have an effect."* I believe there is such a point where consciousness and matter intersect, that this junction exists on a quantum (subatomic) level, and that this extraordinary connection between mind and matter is accessible to us through our love and intent. By harnessing the innate power of our love, we can dynamically and positively activate the body's own healing process. From the DNA to the bones, all cells and systems effortlessly respond to the healing vibration of your love.

The following are some interesting things I want you to know about Quantum-Touch:

Practitioners from each hands-on healing modality who have studied Quantum-Touch in the United States, Canada, and Europe have told me that it significantly increased the power or effectiveness of their healing practice. Chiropractors think of it as an advanced form of chiropractic. Physical therapists think of it as a more effective form of physical therapy. Similarly, acupuncturists have told me that it works like an advanced form of acupuncture. Reiki masters call it *"Reiki empowerment"* or *"turbocharging the Reiki."* Quantum-Touch combines seamlessly with numerous other techniques to enhance their effectiveness: massage, shiatsu, jin shin do, acupressure, polarity, cranial sacral, therapeutic touch, healing touch, and so on.

Quantum-Touch is a wonderful stand-alone therapy for people with no previous training.

This may well be the easiest healing technique that there is to learn. Nearly everyone can learn to do extraordinary healing work after two days of training. It is so easy, you can easily learn from this book. Children can usually learn to do this work almost immediately.

Quantum-Touch will empower people to relieve a tremendous amount of pain and suffering of friends and loved ones. It is truly one of the essential life skills we should all know.

On a purely selfish and personal level, I wish to live in a world where healing is considered real, where healing is universally practiced, and where humanity's kind and generous good nature can be readily expressed. For these and numerous other heartfelt desires, I invite you to join me on a wondrous journey of discovery — the discovery of Quantum-Touch.

> *"It's not important that you know everything – just the important things."*
> — *Miguel de Unamuno*

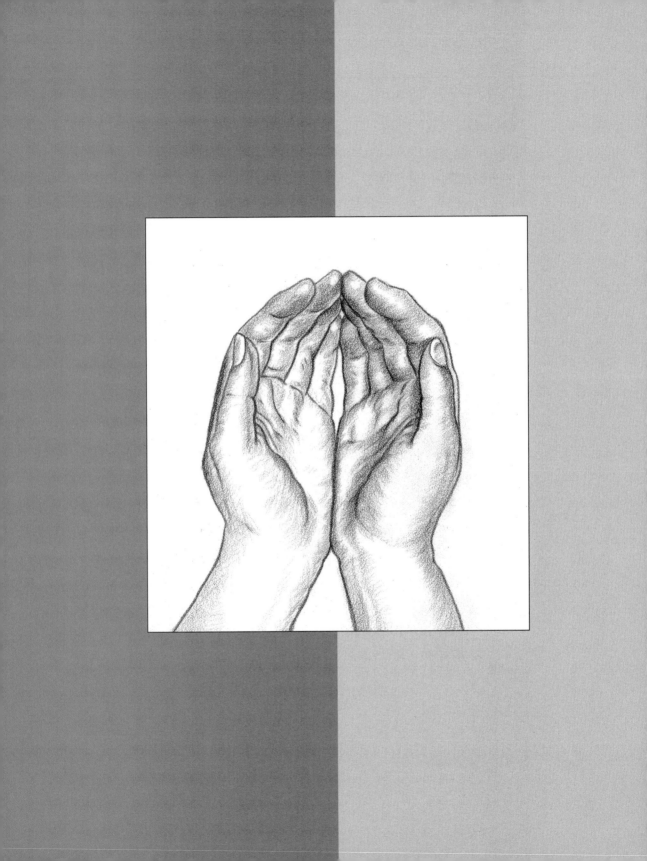

Chapter 1

Discovery

A Hardwired Blessing

Healing is real.
Everyone can do it.
Everyone's love has impact and value.
Your love has impact and value.

The ability to work as a healer is simply a gift. It is a gift within that we need only discover. This ability is ours at birth. It comes as standard equipment on all humans – hardwired into the system.

Café Sessions

"My mother is in a great deal of pain – can she please sit down here?" asked a woman who appeared to be in her sixties. My friend and I, who were looking at a picture book of bats, immediately got off the bench in the bookshop and invited the women to take our seats. The very old woman was bent over and breathing very hard as she painfully and very slowly sat down. I asked the daughter what her mom's problem was, concerned that she might need help. She told me that her mother was having extreme back pain.

For about thirty seconds, I debated within myself as to whether or not I should become involved in this matter, but the "healer" got the best of me. I explained to the daughter that in my profession I use a form of hands-on healing where I very lightly touch the area that is in pain and asked if her mother would like me to do that. She spoke to her mother in French, and the older woman said that that would be fine. In my typical manner, I make wherever I am my office. I have often been seen giving healing sessions at concerts, lectures, movies, golf courses, seminars, supermarkets, or wherever I happen to be. I call these "café sessions."

I asked the mother to point to the spot where her pain was. The daughter translated; and a moment later I was kneeling down with my hands on her mom's painful lower back. She was breathing very hard and her face was contorted by the pain as I began to "run energy" through my hands. Within five minutes, the older woman's face looked peaceful. She turned to me and simply said, "Thank you, I'm all better now." The two women got up, smiled to me, and walked out of the bookstore without another word.

I immediately sat back on the bench and picked up the book, ready to resume where we had left off. To my surprise, my friend was visibly quite shaken by the experience. Although she and I had maintained a casual friendship for a number of years, she had somehow escaped my relentless encounter with people's skepticism. "How can you just pick up the book after an experience like that?" she demanded. I explained that healings are an everyday sort of experience. Although these experiences had been shocking to me when I first began to do Quantum-Touch, over the years I had grown accustomed to them, and had even learned to expect them!

Early Shocks

Over the many years, events like the one previously mentioned have become relatively commonplace for me, but I sometimes forget that to many other people these sorts of happenings can be quite a shock to their system. To be honest, I had more than a few shocks of my own when I first learned to do this sort of work.

When my first book, *Your Healing Hands – The Polarity Experience*, was about to be released in 1978, a friend insisted that I attend a workshop from a remarkable healer. At the beginning of the workshop, I was surprised that the very heavy-set and quiet 60-year-old man who had been sitting by himself and not talking to anyone was the one to be leading the group.

I should tell you that at this particular time in my life, I was feeling pretty cocky about myself, being a young and fit 28-year-old, soon-to-be published author with the first and only popular book on the subject of polarity therapy. Enter Bob Rasmusson, the leader. Bob, a natural storyteller, was absolutely blasé and matter of fact, as he spun out a series of tales that seemed completely incredible to me. Then he asked for one of the members of the audience to act as a volunteer. Up stepped the friend who had invited me to the class.

We took a few minutes as a group to examine my friend's posture. I had never noticed before then that she had a profound "S" curve in her spine: one shoulder was much higher than the other, one hip was higher, and so on. Bob simply worked in the most matter-of-fact way, touching one place, then another. He clearly showed us how her occipital ridge (at the base of the cranium) was severely misaligned. He began taking huge breaths of air and lightly touched the base of her cranium for only a few seconds. Instantly the ridge appeared to be completely even. He touched her hips, touched her shoulders, and ran his hands down her spine. Frankly, I could hardly believe my eyes as I watched bones seeming to melt into place. Within a matter of ten or fifteen minutes, her spine was nearly straight and her hips and shoulders were properly aligned. To put it mildly, I was absolutely astonished!

I immediately came to three major conclusions. The first conclusion was that Bob Rasmusson had some sort of rare and incredible gift. The second conclusion was that no one else would ever be able to learn this. The third conclusion was that I would never be able to learn this. By the end of the day, I found that I was barely able to cause bone positions to move with a light touch. I was stunned. Thankfully, I was wrong on all three counts.

I soon became Bob's friend and neighbor, and would often spend time at his home, observing him working and trying to discover just how and why he was so much more powerful than the people that he trained. For the next couple of years, I would spend hours each day practicing to run the energy. Eventually, I started to get creative in my attempts to do the work, and I was able to discover new ways to amplify the energy and increase my power. I had gotten to a point where Bob liked to have me work on him.

Margery

I think that the single biggest shock I had doing this healing work came about two years after I first learned the basic technique from Bob. I was in Los Angeles and was demonstrating Quantum-Touch before a group of about eight people. Margery had volunteered to be the subject of my demonstration. She had a severe case of osteoporosis and was hunched so far over, she would be looking down at the floor when she walked. I had her put on a button-up shirt backwards so we could get a close look at her back.

I was actually quite shocked when I first saw her spine. Every vertebra was severely misaligned. One vertebra was off far to the left, the next one down was much further to the left and the one below that was somehow pushed massively to the right. Some bones were sticking out further than I could ever have imagined possible. They looked like dinosaur bones. Other bones were indented a great deal. Looking at her spine, it was easy to see why Margery was hunched over when she walked.

I began to run energy into her spine. I would work on one vertebra at a time, spend a minute or two there, and then move down to the next and do the same thing. After about fifteen minutes, people in the group started making comments to the effect, "Is this looking better, or is that my imagination?" Another fifteen or twenty minutes later, I started to hear comments like, "I am pretty sure it is looking better now." It appeared that the bones were gradually finding a more aligned position. After the next fifteen minutes the comments started sounding like, "Oh my God, it is so much better!" By the end of an hour and fifteen minutes, we were all completely amazed.

I could hardly believe my eyes. Every vertebra in Margery's spine was now in a straight line. The vertebrae that were grossly pushed out now appeared to be in a natural position. The vertebrae that were grossly pushed in now appeared to have come out. Margery stood up and suddenly she was much taller than I, when before in her hunched position, we were eye to eye. Margery's daughter came into the room and started crying at the sight of her mother standing up straight. The mother and daughter embraced and cried. The people in the room couldn't stop talking about it, and I was as amazed as any of them.

When I got to my friend's home in Los Angeles where I was staying, the day's events had really thrown my nice and comfortable beliefs into a tizzy. I remember sitting on the floor with my back against the wall contemplating what had just occurred. Suddenly I heard a loud and very believable voice in my own head saying, "THAT DID NOT HAPPEN!" For a brief moment I actually believed it. Then I protested within myself, recalling how people had commented that they thought her spine was gradually looking better, how the vertebrae moved till they were all re-aligned. I recalled how she was standing up very straight and tall, crying gratefully with her daughter. "No," I protested within myself, "it did happen! This is real."

The Bunny

The next shock I encountered was much gentler. My friend Carol had been staying at my home, and since it was near Easter, she brought a baby bunny into my house. When I came home one day, I found that the cute little creature was not in its box and was leaving little brown pellets everywhere. I decided to capture it and put it back into its box. After a minute or two of chasing Mr. Rabbit around the house, I finally had it cornered.

With my hands over its little body, I could feel it trembling in fear, and I wondered what would happen if I started to run energy into it. After about a minute or two of running the energy, I could feel the trembling stop and its little muscles relaxing beneath my hands. Out of curiosity, I kept running the energy. After another couple of minutes the rabbit did something totally unexpected: it stretched its front paws forward as far as it could and its back paws back as far as it could and lay there totally relaxed. "Hey, this is fun," I thought. I kept running energy into the rabbit, and then suddenly the rabbit rolled over on its back with its front paws stretched forward, its back paws back, and my hands on its belly. This bunny looked as if it were having a pleasant day at the beach, all stretched out and drinking in sunlight. I had never seen a rabbit do this nor even heard of a rabbit doing such a thing. At this point I was beginning to get the idea that quite remarkable things could happen during these sessions.

Bob's Gallbladder

One morning, I got a call that Bob Rasmusson had had a gallbladder attack, that he was in a great deal of pain and didn't know any healers in Los Angeles. Would I mind driving down from Santa Cruz (about seven hours) to work on him? I cancelled my plans for the day, and within twenty minutes I was in my car on my way to see Bob.

When I got to Los Angeles, I pulled up to the motel where he was staying and found him in bed. I was told that the doctors wanted to remove his gallbladder. Bob didn't like the idea of being cut open by strangers and having one of his vital organs removed. So I climbed upon his bed, placed my hands over his gallbladder, and went to work running the energy. As you will learn later, this work is very focused and requires a good deal of effort and breathing work on the part of the practitioner. After about an hour and a half, Bob was no longer in pain. He had been sweating a great deal in the latter part of the session. He got out of bed, took a shower, and when he came out he simply said thank you and that he was feeling fine. I drove back to Santa Cruz that evening. I learned thirteen years later the full result of that session. Bob never again had any problems with his gallbladder.

These early "shocks" have served me well in my evolution with Quantum-Touch. Seeing bones suddenly moving back into alignment is something I have learned to take in stride. The big shocks I get now usually come from watching my students do things I have never done before. Now I am not so much surprised as deeply touched by gratitude and wonder.

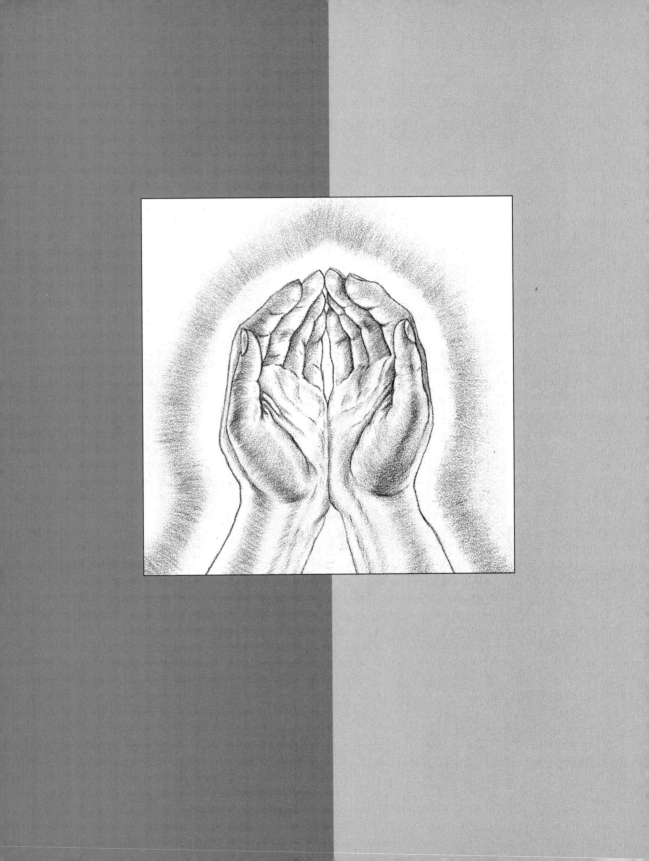

Chapter 2

Resonance, Life-Force, and the Principles of Quantum-Touch

Beneath the surface of our awareness lies a vast
world of vibration. Like water beetles busy
skimming over the top of a lake, we often miss
expansive realms that exist just below the very
waterline of our immediate perception.

Resonance

There truly is a mystery and a wonder in the seemingly simple function of resonance. From the galaxies to the subatomic, all people and particles dance to its power.

If a piano and a guitar were both in tune and a G was played on the piano, the G string on the guitar would also vibrate. Sound waves moving the air are transferring the acoustical energy from the piano to the guitar. Similarly, tuned oscillators, that is, things that can vibrate at the same frequency, require very little work to transfer energy from one to another. In this example, the string on the guitar absorbs the energy waves from the piano because it is tuned to the same frequency. Whenever there are similarly tuned oscillators, they form what is called a resonant system. The guitar and piano string are resonating with one another.

If pendulum-type grandfather clocks were mounted against a wall with their pendulums swinging out of phase to one another, in a matter of days, their pendulums would lock into phase and beat together. In this case, energy transferred through the common wall would be sufficient to allow the clocks to come into phase with one another. This is entrainment, a phenomenon that allows two similarly tuned systems to align their movement and energy so that they match in rhythm and phase. This phenomenon also occurs in the area of electronics. When you have similarly tuned oscillating circuits vibrating at similar frequencies, the slower circuit will rise to match the speed of the faster one. In both of these examples, we can see how energy is transferred from one similarly tuned system to another.

What can we learn from all this? First, when two systems are oscillating at different frequencies, there is an impelling force called resonance that causes the two to transfer energy from one to another. When two similarly tuned systems vibrate at different frequencies, there is another aspect of this energy transfer called entrainment, which causes them to line up and to vibrate at the same frequency. Entrainment is the process by which things align their movement and energy together to match in rhythm and phase.

This seems to work with biological systems as well. On warm nights in many parts of the world, fireflies gathering in a tree will light up at random. Before long, they will all be turning their lights on and off in a coordinated manner. I have often heard crickets or frogs all finding the same rhythm and coordinating their sounds to one another. In these cases, nature finds it useful or perhaps economical to rhythmically entrain the individuals. Perhaps through a more mysterious process, women sharing a house or dormitory over time will find that their menstrual cycles will rhythmically entrain as well. Scientists have found that even disembodied animal hearts, when kept alive in a lab and placed near each other, will entrain – the individual hearts will begin to beat in unison. The process appears to be universal.

Itzhak Bentov may have been absolutely correct in 1977 in his fascinating book Stalking the Wild Pendulum. He states, "We may look at disease as such out-of-tune behavior of one or another of our organs of the body. When a strong harmonizing rhythm is applied to it, the interference pattern of waves, which is the organ, may start beating in tune again." He postulates that this theory may account for the reason energy healing actually works. I agree.

When two things are vibrating at different frequencies through resonance and entrainment, either the lower vibration will come up, the higher vibration will come down, or they will meet in the middle. In Quantum-Touch, practitioners learn through breath and meditation techniques to raise the vibration of their hands to a very high frequency. When they place their hands in proximity to someone else who is in pain, their client's body, like a similarly tuned circuit, will resonate and entrain to the practitioner's hands. Love is the universal vibration that allows people to transfer healing energy from one to another.

In his book, Loving Hands Are Healing Hands, Bruce Berger writes, "Sympathetic resonance describes the tendency of two wave forms with the same degree of arc to vibrate sympathetically together, energizing and communicating universally with each other. Thus wave forms of the same length and frequency will entrain and influence each other throughout all creation. This is the key to understanding one of the dynamics that holds creation together, and to understanding our theory of the body as the energy of sacred sound."

When working with Quantum-Touch, the practitioner holds the highest vibration they can, which becomes the dominant frequency. The "healer" (otherwise known as the client or patient), that is, the person whose body is healing, will simply entrain with and match the vibration of the practitioner. A spiritual teacher named Lazaris has said, "The definition of a great healer is someone who was very sick and got well quickly." In my opinion, anyone who claims to be able to heal others is either ignorant, mistaken, arrogant, or delusional. All they are doing is providing the resonant energy to allow others to heal themselves.

The practitioner simply holds a tremendously strong harmonizing energy, and the client's energy matches that vibration. The innate body intelligence of the person receiving the energy will do whatever the body deems useful to cause healing to occur. The body heals itself with an unfathomable level of intelligence. Western civilization often takes the body's innate healing ability for granted, but it is the true healer. If we look at the cells of our body, we see that we have hundreds of billions of cells that are constantly feeding on oxygen and the food we eat, and releasing carbon dioxide and other waste materials. These cells are also busy reproducing and self-healing, with thousands of microscopic changes taking place every minute of each day! It's a good thing I don't have to keep track of all this activity, since I have a hard enough time just remembering where I left my keys.

Without the breathing and meditative techniques learned in Quantum-Touch, it is actually possible for a practitioner to descend to the vibration of the client and thus become drained from the experience. This does not occur in Quantum-Touch as long as we use the techniques to hold a naturally high resonance.

Perhaps one day, healers will be known as resonant physicians.

Life-Force

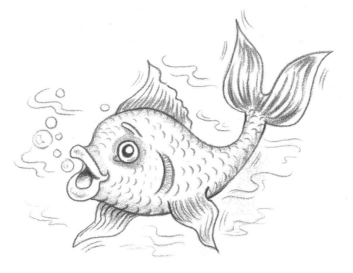

**"No, I have absolutely
no idea what water is,"
said the fish.**

"Why do you ask?"

At every moment, each of us is awash in the perpetual movement of the life-force energy that streams through and around our bodies. Like the fish who has no concept of water, it has only been modern Western cultures who have denied the existence of life-force. According to the rules inherent to the scientific method, everything must be measurable in order to concede its existence. Since scientists do not have sensitive enough instrumentation to measure or prove the existence of life-force, they deny that it is real. This is like denying the existence of a television channel because your set does not receive that station. It is also like denying the existence of love because you can't measure its length or weigh it on a scale.

Life-force is the energy that differentiates that which is living from that which is not. It is the animating current of life, which has been acknowledged, appreciated, and utilized by numerous cultures around the world for thousands of years. The Chinese call it "Chi," and the Japanese call it "Ki." These countries and many others utilize the energy for various healing massage techniques, acupuncture, and numerous forms of martial arts. The Indian yogis have called the energy "Prana" and have used their understanding to achieve higher levels of consciousness through their practices of yoga, pranayama, meditation, and various healing practices. The Hawaiian Kahunas referred to it as "Mana" and also used it for hands-on healing, distant healing, and for prayer.

The irony is that all people actually feel the life-force within them every moment of every day. They just are not aware that they are feeling it. For most of us, the sensations of the life-force energy can be analogous to the background noise of the street where we live. We have grown so completely accustomed to it that we no longer notice it. We only notice the street noise if we stop and pay close attention to it. Sometimes, the most blatant and obvious things are the very last to be seen or acknowledged. Life-force is just such a thing. Yet despite the lack of awareness of life-force, it is easily felt by most individuals without much effort. We just need to know how to look for it.

Perhaps there is a sort of intuitive understanding of the life-force and Prana, even within the English language. When someone dies and their vitality and life-force leaves the body, we say that the person has "expired." Similarly, when someone experiences a wonderful creative flow, we describe them as being "inspired." To "inspire" and "expire" are the same words we use to describe breathing, and the breath happens to be the primary source of Prana.

To summarize, life-force energy is the animating current of life operating with a level of intelligence that boggles human imagination. The life-force permeates all living things.

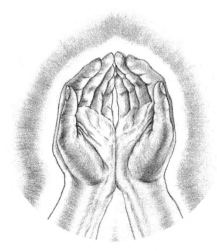

Science of Life-Force Energy

The reality of life-force energy has been well documented by literally thousands of studies. Distant healing and prayer in the laboratory have produced viable and dramatic effects on bacteria, yeasts and other single-celled organisms, as well as on DNA, enzymes and chemicals. Abundant research has also been conducted on plants, animals, and, of course, people.

The fact that this research has not made its way into standard text books and college course work, has, in my opinion, more to do with the politics of science that the validity of the findings. In the words of sociologist, Marcell Truzzi, "Unconventional ideas in science are seldom positively greeted by those benefiting from conformity." If you have an interest in reading about this research, I can suggest the following books:

Energy Medicine: The Scientific Basis
James L. Oschman Churchill
Livingstone, Inc., 2000

Spiritual Healing: Scientific Validation of a Healing Revolution
Daniel Benor
Vision Publications, 2001

Vibrational Medicine
Richard Gerber
Inner Traditions International, Limited 2001

Infinite Mind : Science of Human Vibrations of Consciousness
Valerie V. Hunt
Malibu Publishing Company, 1996

You can also contact the International Society for the Study of Subtle Energies and Energy Medicine, also known as ISSSEEM.
http://www.issseem.org

The True Magic of Touch is Life-Force Energy

For decades, physicians and psychologists have been praising the tremendous value and importance of touch. Studies have shown that babies who are not touched will not grow as quickly as their counterparts who are held regularly. Beyond slow growth, these babies often have weakened immune systems and are more subject to illness. Babies, who are profoundly deficient in their need to be touched, may also suffer severe emotional damage and even violent behavior. Psychology studies have also shown the devastating impact of not being touched in experiments with monkeys taken away from their mothers.

If touch deprivation is abusive, then it stands to reason that abundant touch would be healthy and beneficial. In Jean Liedloff's excellent book, "The Continuum Concept," she discussed how children of the stone age Yequana Indians, living in a "primitive" community in the Brazilian jungle, were held constantly when they were young. As the children grew up, they exhibited no violent behavior. In her two and one half years with this tribe, she realized that children willingly obeyed their elders, and that toddlers played peacefully together without arguing or fighting. Consider that in our "modern" society, it is still a common practice for babies to be separated from their mothers at birth due to medical intervention in maternity wards. These isolated babies hear nothing but the crying of other newborns. Away from the arms of their mothers, they cry themselves to sleep.

The question I am raising is this: What is touch, and what makes it so important? If touch were merely physical contact, a mechanical rocker and a moving piece of rabbit fur could provide a baby's touch needs. But I do not believe that the value of touch is merely physical. I believe that it is much more than just the mechanics of being stroked. In my opinion, the true value of touch is the life-force energy ^ and the love - in that touch.

This came more clearly to my awareness this year with the case of Teddy, a baby who was born 13 weeks premature. Teddy was the seventh child born to a woman who had been an alcoholic for 10 years. He was diagnosed with severe fetal alcohol syndrome, tested positive for crack cocaine, and the baby's doctor said that he "saw no real hope" for this boy. At the time of his birth, Teddy could not move any muscles and would lie helplessly, like a tiny limp bag of bones. His eyes were tightly closed and his mouth didn't have the muscles to suck from a bottle. He was only sufficiently developed to be able to swallow. Teddy was so tiny that his whole hand was smaller than a man's thumbnail. After two weeks in the hospital, Teddy was released into a foster home where the adoptive father, mother and all five children all knew how to use Quantum-Touch. Everyone in the house ran energy for Teddy. (Keep in mind you only need one person to be effective, though it is more fun with seven.)

When Teddy became stronger and could cry for food in the morning, Michael, the father, would pick up the baby and run energy into his tiny body. Amazingly, Teddy would stop squirming and crying within a few seconds, and become completely relaxed in Michael's hands. After receiving Quantum-Touch, Teddy would sit quietly and wait patiently for his food formula as it was being prepared. This response is highly reminiscent of the story of the frightened bunny in chapter one that flipped over on its back, or of Henri's turtle, in chapter eleven, that would rest for an hour with its head and limbs outside the shell while being held.

When Teddy got older and it was time for his vaccinations, all the other children screamed as needles punctured both thighs. Michael simply put a hand on Teddy's chest and ran energy. To the surprise of the nurse, Teddy didn't cry at all. On the third round of vaccinations six months later, Michael experimented and lifted his hand off Teddy's chest after the second inoculation. Teddy immediately started to turn purple and began to cry. Michael placed his hand back on the chest and within a few seconds, Teddy took a big sigh and became relaxed again.

Today Teddy, or little "Boo Boo," as he has come to be called, is a source of amazement. His doctor who once "saw little hope for normal development" has proclaimed that he is developmentally normal, and that he can't believe this is the same baby. At 10 months old, all of Teddy's developmental indicators are within normal range and age appropriate. He is at 100% on the developmental grading, and is of average weight for a child his age. The facial morphology has significantly normalized. In the words of Dr. Norman Shealy, M.D., in a recent conversation, "I would love to see every premature, sick or addicted baby be treated with Quantum-Touch." Perhaps one day that will happen. I believe that it is only a matter of time.

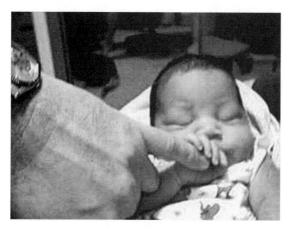

Teddy at 3 weeks of age (left)

Teddy at 10 months (below)

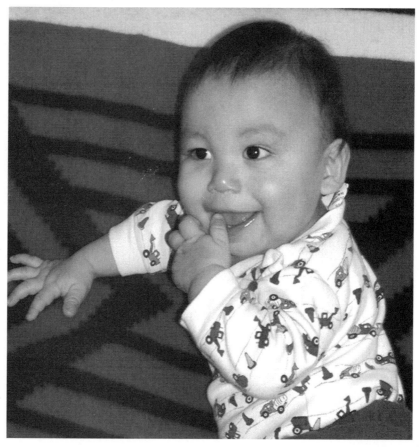

Quantum-Touch Principles

- Love is a universal vibration; love communicates to all species, functions on all levels and expresses our true nature. It is the foundation of all healing and the core essence of the life-force.

- The ability to assist in healing is natural to all people.

- Healing is a skill that can be taught and that grows stronger with practice. Practitioners become stronger at running the energy and in their healing ability over time.

- Energy follows thought. The practitioner uses intention and various meditations to create a high-energy field and uses that field to surround the area to be healed.

- Resonance and entrainment cause the area being healed to change its vibration to match that of the practitioner. The practitioner simply raises and holds the new resonance.

- No one can really heal anyone else. The person in need of healing is the healer. The practitioner simply holds a resonance to allow the body to heal itself.

- Trusting the process is essential. The work may cause temporary pain or other distressing symptoms that are all part of the healing. The life-force and the healing process work with complexity and wisdom that are beyond our conception and comprehension.

- The energy follows the natural intelligence of the body to do the necessary healing. The practitioner pays attention to "body intelligence" and "chases the pain."

- The practitioner is also receiving a healing by doing the work.

- Breathing amplifies the life-force.

- Combining breathing and meditation techniques together causes the energy to line up, which increases its power many times, like a laser.

- Synergy is the effect of multiple healers working together and is greater than the sum of the parts. It can be very powerful.

- Each person's gifts in life and in healing are unique. Some people are especially gifted at treating specific conditions.

- Healing can be accomplished from a distance and can be highly effective.

- Quantum-Touch combines easily and effectively with other healing modalities.

- The ability to connect with one's spirituality, in whatever form it is perceived to be, and asking for help adds another dimension of power to this work.

Many of these principles will be expanded in later chapters of this book.

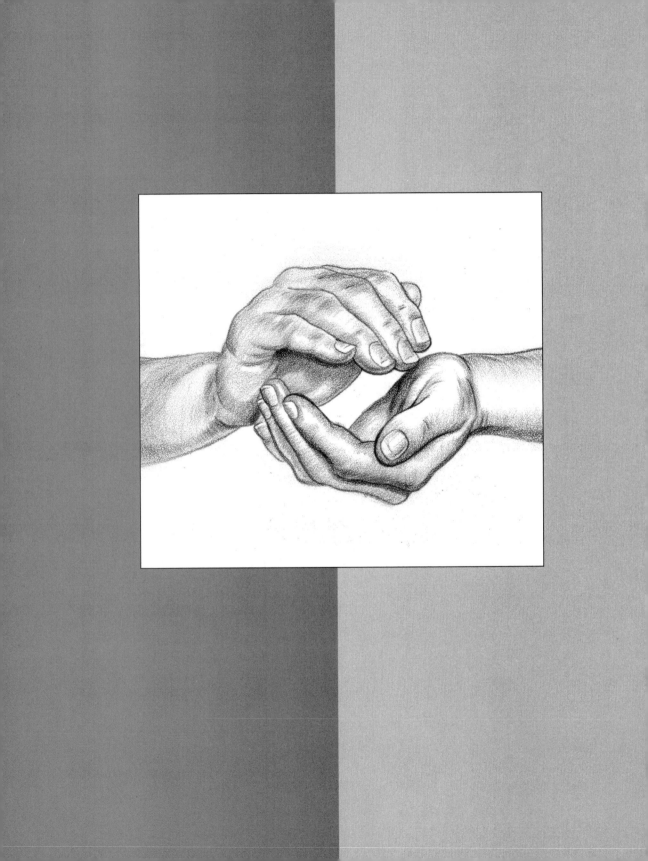

Chapter 3

Healing Hands

"I think that the best kind of medicine
is the gentlest treatment that produces
the maximum healing response."

– Andrew Weil, M.D.

Healing and Chopsticks

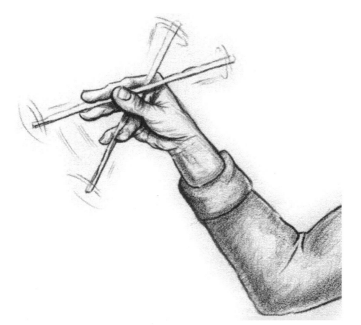

Far simpler than learning to read,
as natural as learning to hug those you love,
healing is probably the easiest skill that you will ever learn.

For many people, learning to heal with your hands is far easier
than learning to use chopsticks.

To Be a "Healer"

There are those who would have us believe that it takes many years of hard work and discipline to become healing practitioners. They would have us believe that only the most brilliant, gifted, and extensively trained among us could ever hope to obtain such a title. If the truth be told, children, seniors, and everyone in between can learn to be healing practitioners. I would even go so far as to say that physicians and people with postgraduate degrees can learn to do this healing work.

There have been many acclaimed "healers" whose talents have been well documented and accepted as genuine. However, most of them had no explanation for what they were doing or how it was occurring. The significance of Quantum-Touch is that we now have a cognitive explanation for how to stimulate the healing process, and we have a proven methodology for instructing others how to do this successfully as well.

Since the true healer is the person receiving the energy, the practitioner is merely acting as the catalyst to allow the healer to heal him or herself, and to access and utilize a higher vibrational field of energy. During this process, the truth about healing is as follows:

- Healing is real.

- Becoming a highly effective healing practitioner is one of the easiest skills to learn.

- Healing is a great and tremendous joy.

- Anyone with a strong desire can learn this.

- You can learn to be an extraordinary healing practitioner, starting now!

It Starts with Love

Healing work is all about love, and the practitioner learns to hold a vibratory field of this love. To clarify my terms, when I say "love," I am not speaking in the traditional sense of the sort of love that a mother has for a child, a husband for a wife, or about a winged cherub with a bow and arrow. I'm speaking of a more basic form of love – one that is more innate and intrinsic.

Have you ever watched children play? They seem to always say, "Watch me!" So whether you are from the child's culture or any other culture, whether you speak the language or not, if you sit there simply watching that child, he or she will feel loved. Simply giving your attention to a child is automatically experienced as an act of loving. This is what I call nonenculturated or nonassociative love because it has nothing to do with your background, your race, religion, politics, or other beliefs you may hold. Quantum-Touch is about being present, which is an expression of your essence.

I would call this kind of love "preconditional" and believethat your very nature and essence is made up of the fabric of love. Whether you believe it is there or not (in my opinion) is irrelevant. This love is the essential nature of your being that comes through your hands regardless of your mood. Your fundamental, instinctive, and most basic energy is that of love. You don't have to work at it – it is who you are. As a rock does not have to try to be more "rocklike" and water does not have to try to be wetter, we do not have to try to have more essence of love. We can, however, endeavor to acknowledge how much love there really is.

Intent is something that happens so automatically, most people just miss it. When you simply walk across the room, you already generated the intention to do so. You see, love and intention are among the most natural qualities we have. So don't worry. If you are reading this book to learn to do healing, you already have sufficient love and intention to do a wonderful job.

Basic Energy Exercises

Quantum-Touch is powerful healing work. In order to do Quantum-Touch, it is necessary to first learn various energy exercises. Most people will find these exercises easy to learn and highly pleasurable to do. However, you need to take your time and practice these techniques thoroughly. These exercises are designed to help you increase your awareness of life-force energy and physical sensations in your hands. The extra time and effort you spend with them will make a huge difference in your ability to run the energy and increase the power of your healing sessions. Eventually, you will feel a growing sense of mastery, and they will become second nature to you.

The energy exercises are placed in a particular order that will facilitate your learning and utilization of these skills. Once you have completed the first round of energy exercises, you will be ready to learn the basic breathing techniques. At that point, you will be able to start combining the breathing and energy exercises together to start doing your healing work.

If you put forth your best effort while working with these exercises, your success will grow. The best approach is to concentrate while maintaining a very relaxed frame of mind. The less muscle tension you hold in your body and hands, the better you will do.

Exercise 1: Feel Your Finger

1. Hold a finger in the air and spend about two minutes or more feeling as much sensation in your finger as you can. Tune into the sensation in your finger and focus on intensifying your awareness.

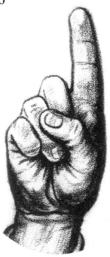

2. Feel how the skin wraps around your finger. See if you can feel the blood as it moves through your finger. Use your imagination and see if you can feel how your fingernail sits on your finger. Try to feel sensation under your fingernail. The key is to use your focused attention to feel your finger completely.

The basic premise is that energy follows thought. Wherever you place your attention, energy follows. By increasing the sensations in your finger by moving and holding energy there, you are causing physiological changes to occur as well. These sensations may seem like ordinary sorts of feelings you have in your body, but as you will see, you are actually sensing life-force energy. Most people will say that they can feel a tingling sensation in their finger. Some people describe the feeling as vibrating, buzzing, carbonated, or hot. Since everyone experiences things differently, people are likely to use different words. Some people describe the energy as heat, throbbing, thickness, heaviness, or simply as an increased awareness of the finger itself.

Sensing the life-force energy is not something foreign to us. Rather, the life-force is an energy we have always felt but have just not learned to identify. If you are alive, and since you are reading this I'll assume you are, you have been feeling it every minute of every day.

If you don't feel any of these sensations, try imagining that you are stroking your finger with a feather. Stroke your finger back and forth with this imaginary feather. Now pay close attention to whatever sensation you do feel in your finger. Take about a minute or so to feel any sensation. This sensation may not seem like much, and you may be using a word to describe it that I have not used, but whatever it is, I suggest you use that sensation as a starting point to experience the energy. If you are not able to feel any sensation in your finger, I suggest that you work with the other exercises and see if you can generate sensation in other parts of your body.

When doing the exercise, some of you may feel your whole hand tingling or even other parts of your body as well. If this occurs, this is OK, and it means you are doing wonderfully well. You are already starting to do the next exercise spontaneously.

Exercise 2: Feeling Your Body Parts

In this exercise we will bring energy and sensation to all parts of your body. The sensations you feel will probably be similar to those you experienced in your finger in the previous exercise.

Many of you will find that there may be places in your body where it seems difficult or even impossible to feel any sensation, no matter how much attention you focus there. This is usually a temporary problem, and it is quite common and nothing to worry about in terms of doing a great job running energy. The more you practice, the easier it becomes to feel all parts of your body.

This exercise is best done with the help of a friend.

1. Take your shoes off, and then while sitting or lying down, have your friend lightly stroke upward, from your feet to your ankles, for a few seconds. The touch should cover as much surface area as possible on the feet and ankles in a gentle sweeping motion like petting a cat, for only about one or two seconds. After this upward stroke, your friend should let go and not be touching you.

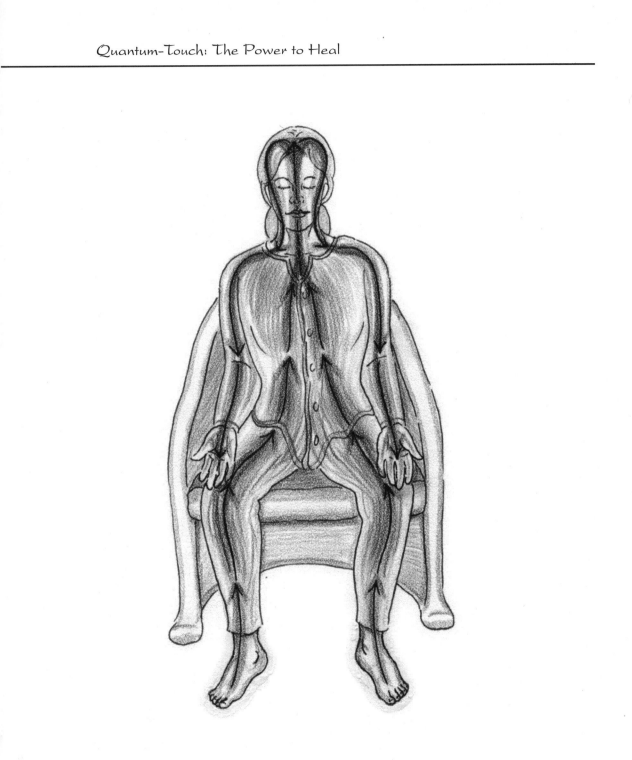

The purpose of this exercise is to assist you in being able to feel as much sensation as possible in your feet and ankles. Ideally, you will feel your feet with the same level of intensity that you felt in your finger earlier. Having the touch of a friend is useful in helping you focus your attention. Letting go is also an essential part of the exercise because it allows you to feel the sensations in your body yourself without being touched. If you cannot generate sensation in your feet, ask your friend to stroke them again. If you still can't feel anything, ask your friend to move on to the next step.

2. When you are ready, and you are feeling these sensations well, have your friend place her hands on the area just above the ankles for a couple of seconds moving upwards towards your shins, and then let go.

3. Continue on up the rest of the body, stroking shins, knees, thighs, hips, lower pelvis, stomach, chest, neck, and up to the head. Then come down from the head to the shoulders, arms, and hands. This pattern of stroking from toe to head is useful for stimulating the directional flow of the energy when you are running the energy throughout your body and when you are doing a healing session. We will do the back of the body later.

4. When you are finished feeling the energy flowing throughout your body, change places with your friend and use the same techniques to give them the experience also.

5. If you are doing this alone, touch your own feet and sweep upwards for about two to five seconds and then let go. Feel as much sensation as you can and repeat the upward sweeping as many times as necessary. Since another person's touch is less predictable than your own, you may have to use a little more attention and focus when working alone. Continue stroking up the body towards the head, then down the shoulders, arms, and end with the hands.

Some people simply have a more difficult time being able to experience sensations in their body. If this applies to you and you are unable to feel a particular part of your body, just move on to another part of your body that you can feel. (Simply repeating this exercise will assist you to clear the blocked areas over time.) The more you repeat this exercise, the more easily you will be able to feel sensations throughout your body. You may discover that parts of your body where you had felt nothing before are now readily experiencing sensation.

Most people report that this exercise causes highly pleasurable body sensations. So enjoy. (Who said learning to heal had to be painful?)

What to Do If You Can't Feel Body Sensation Anywhere

I have found that one or two percent of the people I teach are kinesthetically impaired. That is, they have difficulty feeling any sensation whatsoever in their body. I have found that these people can still learn to do this, but it requires more effort and concentration than for someone who has access to full body sensations.

If you find that you cannot feel any body sensation, try holding your attention inside the parts of the body that are being stroked. In time, sensation will awaken. Admittedly this is not easy, but with practice, I have found that most people will be able to start generating sensation. You will still be able to do the healing work, but it may require more concentration as well.

Exercise 3: 18 Inch Sweeps

1. We will be following the same pattern of gentle sweeping strokes that we used in the last exercise. This time, however, have your friend use longer sweeps, about 18 inches in length. Once again, the touch is light (your friend is doing no healing here) and the touch lasts for two to five seconds. Have your friend use a sweeping touch from the feet all the way up to the knees. This

stroke should also take about one or two seconds to complete. Use your attention and intention to bring your sensation to that area, and then tell your friend to either repeat the motion or to proceed.

2. The purpose of touching in longer sweeps is to more fluidly and consciously move the energy throughout your body. We are creating a smooth wave of energy flowing throughout our bodies. After your friend has let go, feel the sensations in your body as strongly as you can. The object is to get these areas of your body tingling, vibrating, buzzing, or getting hot, as you did in the first exercise. If you do not feel any sensation, or would like to have the touch repeated, ask your friend to touch you again. Be sure to wait until you are ready before moving on to the next position. After your friend has completed the process, you can trade places and repeat the process.

3. If you are doing this alone, lightly stroke yourself from the feet to the knees for a few seconds and stop to feel sensations. Feel as much sensation as you can. Repeat the stroke if you are not feeling any sensations. Gradually work your way up to the head, then down the shoulders and into the hands.

Blocked Areas

If you have trouble feeling a particular area, you can ask your friend to touch that place again to help you to feel it. If you can't bring sensation to the area after three tries, don't worry about it, move on to the next area. In time that area of your body will "wake up" and be able to feel the energy. In most cases people learn to wake up difficult areas within hours or perhaps weeks. In rare cases, it may take a year or more to do this. Note that this does not significantly affect your power or effectiveness when it comes to doing great Quantum-Touch sessions.

Exercise 4: Full Body Sweeps on Front and Back

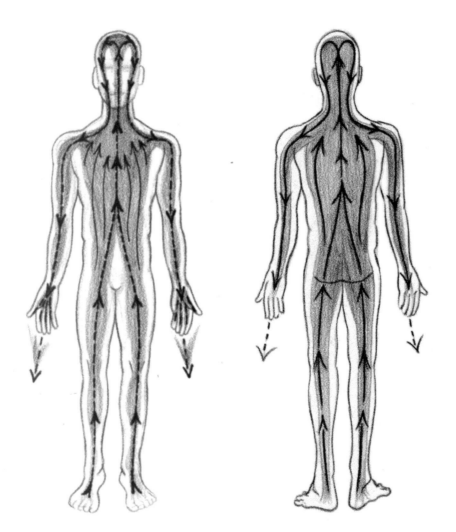

One Large Stroke up the Front

With one large stroke, go up from the feet, up the legs, up the torso and the top of the head, down the neck, over the shoulders and down the arms, and into the hands. The entire stroke should take about two seconds to complete.

If you are receiving the touch, give yourself time to recreate the experience and bring as much sensation throughout your body as possible. Go ahead and ask your friend to repeat the large stroke a time or two, each time allowing your body time to recreate the sensation. Do this until it becomes easy to bring about whole body sensation with the power of intention and attention.

If you are doing this on yourself, you can stroke up your feet, legs, torso to the head, cross your arms, and stroke down each arm.

One Large Sweep up the Back

In this exercise, we follow the same pattern as the sweeps on the front of the body, except we are sweeping the back as well. With your friend standing, make one long continuous sweep up from their feet to the top of their head and down the shoulders, arms, and into the hands. If you are working by yourself, this step will not be as easy or as fluid. Just do your best. Sweeping the back is not a crucial step.

Feel the sensation as strongly as you can in each part of your body. If you want your friend to repeat any of the sweeps, ask them to do so. Otherwise, say "OK" when you are ready for them to move on to the next area.

Energy Exercise 5:
Full Body Sweep Using Your Mind

In this step, you mentally recreate the sensations of the full body sweeps. With the power of your imagination, see yourself receiving a full body sweep. Now let yourself feel the tingling, vibrating, or other sensations throughout your body, and feel those sensations as strongly as you can. Allow the sensations to flow through your body in the same pattern as before: from your feet, up through your legs, up your torso, down your head, and out your arms into your hands. This pattern of moving energy from the feet to the top of your body and then down your arms into your hands is what I will refer to as a full body sweep.

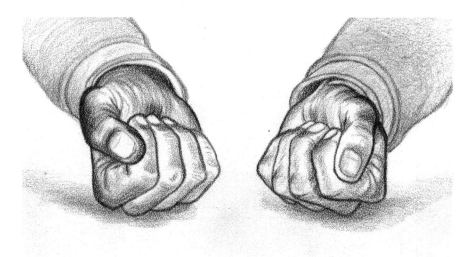

Take your hands and close them into very loose fists. Now direct the energy in your body into your hands. Notice how much sensation is in your hands now. Try this with your hands closed into the loose fist position and with your hands open.

Summary

Now that you have completed the first set of exercises for running energy, let's take a look at what has happened here.

First, you have learned to bring attention and sensation to any part of your body. If there are still places that you cannot bring sensation into with your focused attention, keep practicing and they will open up for you. It is not necessary that you have every place open and "tingling" to do a great job of healing. Do your best, and you will continue to improve.

If you have done these exercises, you are most likely at the point where you no longer need to have anyone touch you to help you awaken the process within yourself. You will be capable of bringing those sensations to your awareness yourself.

You can practice running energy almost any time, anywhere – for example, standing in line at a bank or grocery store, while talking on the phone, at a boring business meeting, or while watching TV or a movie. Since the experience is so pleasurable, I recommend that you practice this exercise often.

As you continue to practice this exercise, you should discover that you will become significantly stronger at running the energy. Repeat these exercises as needed and learn to bring the energy more intensely into each area of your body and direct it into your hands.

Basic Breathing Techniques

In all the Quantum-Touch work, it is important to use the breathing techniques 100 percent of the time in 100 percent of your sessions. If you were in my class, I would be telling you this over and over again during the times that you were practicing running the energy.

Breathing techniques are an essential and crucial part of running energy. Breathing amplifies the power of the life-force, and its value cannot be overstated. The Indian yogis called the life-force in the air we breathe "Prana." The Hawaiian kahunas experienced the life-force in the breath and called it "Mana." They considered it an essential factor in the process of prayer and healing. I find it interesting and somewhat amusing that the early Hawaiians were dumbfounded and amazed when they saw the Western priests suddenly drop down to their knees and pray without doing any special breathing whatsoever. The word *haole*, which refers to these visitors from the mainland, actually means without breath.

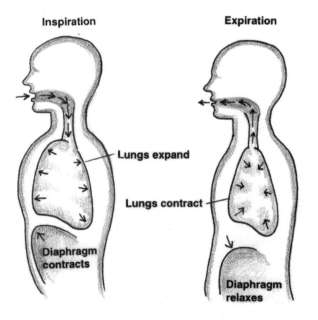

Most people are shallow breathers. Most common are the "upper chest" breathers. You know who you are; you tend to draw shallow breaths into your upper chest. Other shallow breathers are "stomach" breathers. They (myself included) tend to take shallow breaths in the area of the stomach.

Every one of the Quantum-Touch breathing techniques require full breaths. Breathe through your nose unless the sheer volume of air makes it easier for you to breathe through your mouth. Quantum-Touch works quite well with mouth or nose breathing. A full breath begins below the belly button and pushes the belly out on the inhalation. When the lungs are full, the breath should lift the shoulders slightly. Practice taking some full breaths now. Place your hands over your tummy, below the navel, and inhale, feeling your hands being pushed away on the inhalation. Bring the breath all the way up to the top of the shoulders so they raise slightly. This may feel uncomfortable for a while to people who are not accustomed to deep breathing.

Breathing Techniques

1. The 4-4 Breath

The 4-4 breath has become a favorite breathing technique for many of my students. As you inhale to the count of four, do a very thorough full body sweep from your feet to the top of your head. Be sure to feel as much sensation as you can, as you bring your awareness all the way through your body. On the exhalation, let all the sensation you can generate surge into your hands as strongly as possible. This is an easy breathing pattern, but it takes a lot of concentration to do it well.

2. The 1-4 Breath

The 1-4 is an extremely powerful boosting technique. Here you take in a complete breath to the count of one and exhale completely to the count of four. Inhaling to the count of one requires a very strong effort and mouth breathing. Back off if you start to get dizzy.

3. Fire Breathing Followed by 2-6 or 1-4

This is the most powerful of the breaths for boosting the energy and can be done as often as one time every minute. Overuse of this breath can cause fainting. Back off from this technique if you start feeling faint. (Do not use this technique while driving or operating heavy machinery.) Rapidly blow out and pull in large amounts of air five to seven times. Your lungs work like large bellows moving a great volume of air. You can imagine you are blowing out a candle that is two feet from you on the exhalation and then on the inhalation, you are pulling back in all the air you just exhaled. The inhalation and exhalation require mouth breathing and are very rapid, like fast panting, taking only a few seconds to complete the five to seven breaths. Once you have completed the rapid inhalation and exhalation, then immediately take in a very full inhalation and exhale for four counts or six, and then continue with techniques 1 or 2.

4. The 2-6 Breath

This is a very powerful breathing technique for boosting the energy during your Quantum-Touch sessions. The name says it all: two counts for the inhalation and six counts for the exhalation. A count is about one second in length.

This breath requires a bit of effort. You have to really pull in a good deal of air to fill your lungs with a complete breath in just two counts. There is no holding of the breath in this or any other technique. The exhalation is smooth and even to the count of six.

Connecting the Energy to Your Breathing

Now that you have moved the energy throughout your body and have practiced the basic breathing techniques, it is time to practice combining these elements together. I use the term "running energy" to describe the process of linking body awareness exercises with the breathing techniques. In Quantum-Touch, it is the combination of the breathing with the movement of energy that causes the system to work so effectively.

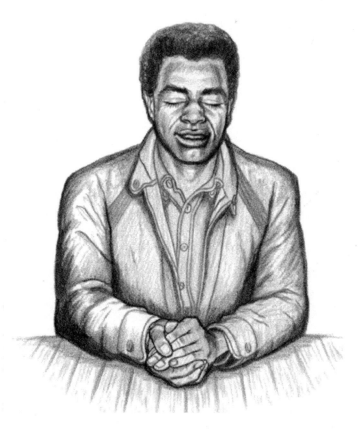

1. Sitting or standing, mentally do a full body sweep on yourself (see p.36). The key is to feel as much sensation move through your entire body as you possibly can. Having practiced the previous exercises, most people are now able to use the power of

their intention well enough to generate sensation through much or all of their body. Cup your hands together or gently close your hands to form "loose fists." Do two or three full body sweeps and feel the energy gather in your hands. Once you can feel the sensations increase in your hands, it is time to coordinate it with the breathing.

2. Start a 2-6 breathing pattern. Take full breaths to the count of two, with a full exhalation to the count of six, and place all your attention in your hands. Feel the energy building on the exhalation. Do this for a few minutes as you coordinate the exhalation with the sensation. Always work to increase sensation on the exhalation throughout these exercises. Don't worry about feeling the energy build in your hands on the inhalation. Focus on the six counts of exhalation. If you are doing this correctly, you will feel an increase of sensation in your hands.

3. With the hands still gently closed or cupped, start the 1-4 breathing pattern. Notice how the sensations in your hands change as you do this. Work to feel the sensations increase on the exhalation. This simply requires that you keep your attention in your hands and have the intention to increase the sensations. Developing the ability to increase sensation and tie it to the breath is one of the most important skills of Quantum-Touch. If you are doing this correctly, you should notice that the sensation in the hands has grown by changing the tempo of your breath. As long as you don't get yourself dizzy and fall over, the more air you are moving, the more the life-force will increase.

4. Start doing the fire breathing technique. Again, your hands should be gently closed or cupped as you do the breathing. Once you have finished the rapid inhalations and exhalations, take a large inhalation and go into a 1-4 or 2-6 breathing pattern. Now notice how the sensations in your hands have changed. If you feel an increase in sensations on the exhalations, you are doing a great job and are ready for the next step. The next step is doing a healing session.

Putting This All Together

The time has come to try out your new found skills. At this point, most people can generate some sensation in their hands, do full body sweeps, and are able to do the breathing fairly well. In addition, most people are able to put these elements together and feel the increase in sensation in their hands. Here is the surprise: most are not aware of just how powerfully they can now assist another person who is in pain with just these rudimentary skills.

It doesn't even seem to matter if you are disbelieving or skeptical of this last statement. The fact that you can change the vibration in your hands will create an energy field that can assist in healing and alleviating pain. Through practice and experience you can discover the power of healing energy and gain confidence in your ability.

The next section will give you a few tips on how to work with what you have just learned. More detailed information regarding these instructions will follow.

Your First Healing Session

1. Find someone you know who is experiencing pain. Ask your friend how much pain or discomfort he or she is feeling. Have your friend rate their discomfort on a scale from 1 to 10, where 10 is the worst. It is amazing how many times people forget how bad the pain was after it is gone.

2. Ask your friend where they hurt. The most important thing is that you do not make any assumptions about where their pain is located. If you ask someone where he is hurting, and he says that his left shoulder hurts, you will still need to ask him which part

of the shoulder it is that hurts. Unless you are truly psychic, your assumptions are often wrong in this matter. The best way to find out exactly where your friend is experiencing pain is to ask and have him point it out or place your hands in the right place for you. This is what I have come to call the "Where does it hurt?" technique.

3. Be sure to place your hands either directly over or on either side of, the areas in which your friend is experiencing pain. By "sandwiching" the area of pain between your hands, you are in effect creating a strong resonant field that will allow that tissue to change vibration and heal itself.

4. If you are working on a problem with someone's back or neck, place one hand on each side of the vertebrae of the spine.

5. Experiment with the breathing techniques, paying close attention to any sensations in your hands on the exhalation. Be sure to take large breaths the entire time that you are working. If you start feeling a little dizzy, back off a bit.

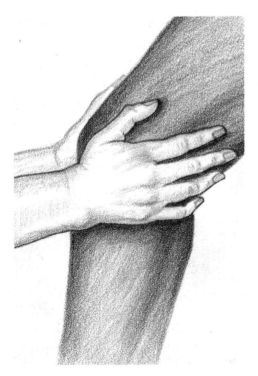

6. Make sure that your hands are relaxed, as energy will flow more easily out of hands that are loose and open. Always remember to use both hands during a session. This helps you generate a better field into or through the tissue. **While you are working, pay close attention to how the sensations in *your* hands change.**

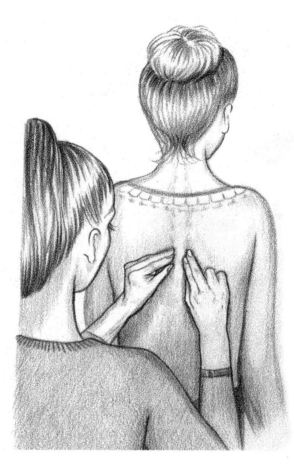

This will prove to be very useful information that I will discuss shortly.

7. "Chase" the pain. Ask your friend to keep you informed if the sensations in their body shift or change. It is quite common for someone to report that pain has moved, or that they are experiencing more sensation somewhere else. When this occurs, move your hands to that place. In this manner, it is as if we are "chasing the pain."

8. Leave your hands in place for twenty to thirty minutes or more, if pain has not subsided.

9. At the end of your session, ask them to rate their pain again.

Understanding the Sensations You Feel in Your Hands During a Healing Session

Quantum-Touch practitioners are likely to experience a wide variety of sensations in their hands. It is important to pay close attention to these sensations, as they will often give you valuable clues about what is happening in the session and what to do next. The intensity of the sensations that you feel is a direct indicator of how much of the energy that you have generated is being received from your healing touch. The more open their body is to the energy you are generating, the stronger the sensations will feel.

The Five Basic Patterns to the Energy

There are five primary patterns of energy you are likely to feel in your hands when you are doing Quantum-Touch work:

1. **The Blocked Pattern –** Feeling very little in your hands to begin with, and then sensations gradually building to a peak. Very blocked areas are often areas of chronic problems, of diseased organs, or sometimes of acute pain (but not often).

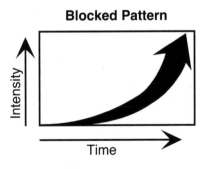

When you are working on an area that is very blocked, you are likely to feel very little in your hands. However, in most cases, the longer you hold your hands there, the more you will notice that the energy is slowly and surely building up. This can take time to happen. You may leave your hands in one position for ten, twenty, forty minutes, or even an hour. Over time, the energy in your hands will gradually feel stronger and stronger until it seems to reach a peak of intensity. Sometimes the sensation of energy will stay at that peak level for a long time and suddenly rise to plateau at an even greater degree of intensity. More often, the energy begins to level out at some point, and then it may go down slightly.

2. **The Common Pattern** – Feeling a moderate amount of sensation in your hands, which builds to a peak and then diminishes. This is the pattern you will probably encounter most of the time.

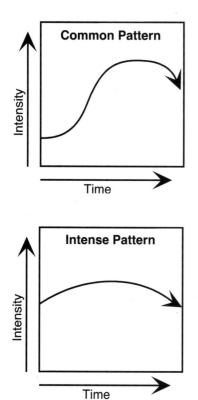

Sometimes, the sensation of energy that you feel will build to a very high pitch where it seems to plateau. At that point, it is often a good idea to use some fire breathing to see if you can raise it to an even higher level. As you work to run the energy and increase its intensity, eventually you will find that it levels out or goes down. When that occurs, it may well be time to move your hands to another place.

3. **The Intense Pattern** – Feeling very strong energy in your hands, which eventually diminishes over time. This pattern is most often felt when working with acute symptoms, or with a person whose body, for whatever reason, is highly receptive to the energy. It looks like this:

Being aware of the sensations in your hands and the patterns that energy work typically follows can help you determine how long to hold your hands in any particular position. You can also simply ask your friend how he or she is feeling. When all the pain is gone or has greatly diminished, it is usually a good indication that the job is done for now.

4. **The Full Pattern** – Sometimes when you are running the energy, everything seems to be working fine, and then at some point during the session, you may discover that you feel nothing in your hands. When you pull your hands away, your hands will feel a great deal of tingling. This is an indication of the Full Pattern.

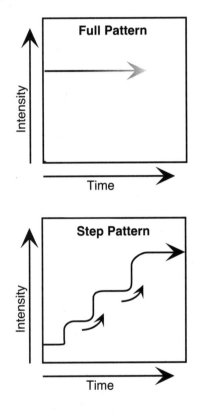

The full pattern occurs when the person has absorbed as much energy as their body wants to absorb. At this point you have no more sensations in your hands when you touch the person. If you come back in ten or twenty minutes, their body may be able to resonate to a higher vibration and "take in" more energy.

5. **The Step Pattern** – Sometimes when you are running energy, you may feel that the intensity has peaked. At this point, if you do some fire breathing, you may discover that your hands are now vibrating at an even higher frequency. Just when you think that the energy has peaked and will go no higher, doing the fire breath again may cause the energy to go up again and again, like climbing steps. Eventually, the energy truly levels out, goes down, or sensation disappears from your hands, and you know that you are done.

The awareness of these patterns is not rocket science. You are not going to hurt a person by putting too much energy in, and if you don't complete the healing, the person will tell you that there is more to be done. The important thing is to enjoy yourself and to be there for the person you are working on.

Static Energy

Most of the time when you give Quantum-Touch sessions, your hands will feel quite normal. By using the breathing techniques I have described, practitioners are naturally protected from allowing their energy to match the vibration of the person they are working on. On occasion, you may feel a sort of "static energy" that can accumulate on your hands. This static energy can be easily released by simply rinsing the hands, wrists, and forearms in cool water after each session. You can feel this energy as a thickness around your hands, as if you were wearing "energy gloves." The sensation is not particularly uncomfortable, but it is recommended that you wash your hands at the earliest opportunity. For many people, the washing of the hands at this point brings a very real sense of relief. Shaking your hands as if to shake off water does the same thing, but in my experience, it doesn't seem to work as well as rinsing the hands with cool water. I find the need to rinse the hands minimally important with Quantum-Touch. When I practiced polarity therapy, I found it to be vitally important from an energy standpoint. Washing the hands is also an excellent thing to do for hygienic purposes.

Some of my students who are polarity therapy and Reiki practitioners have told me that they have felt drained after doing polarity or Reiki sessions. **The trick is to always use the breathing techniques throughout the sessions.** One friend who practices Reiki and had learned Quantum-Touch was trading sessions with me for a while. One day she complained that she felt energy backing up her arm. I asked her if she had stopped the breathing, and sure enough, she had. When I reminded her to keep using the breathing techniques, the problem immediately disappeared.

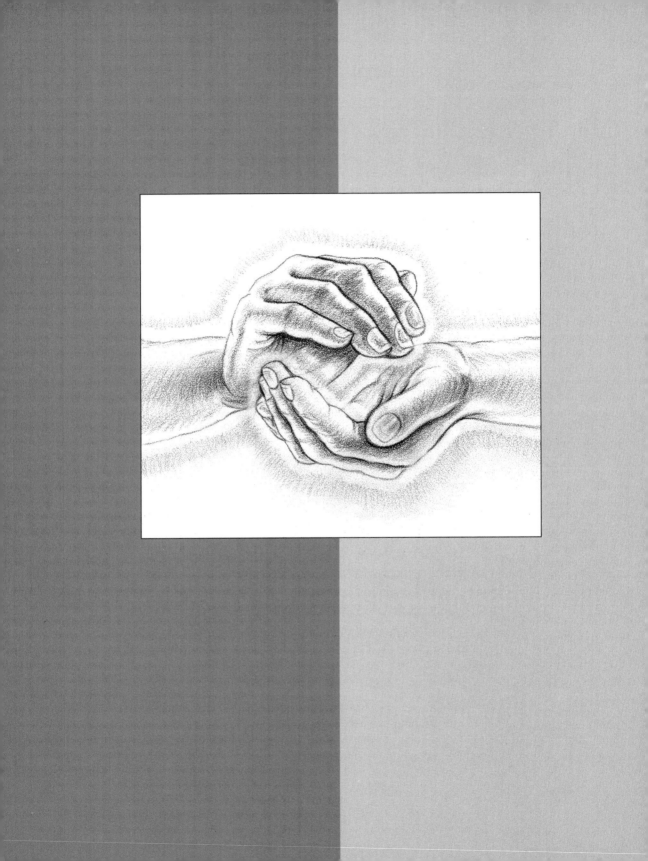

Chapter 4

Frequently Asked Questions

"Life is not a problem to be solved
but a mystery to be experienced."

– Frank Herbert

Over the many years that I have been teaching Quantum-Touch workshops, I seem to be asked many of the same questions again and again. So in my own way of including you in one of my classes, I am providing you with a question-and-answer chapter. For your convenience, the questions have been divided into various general topics. Enjoy.

Practicing Quantum-Touch Techniques

Do you get stronger with practice?

Yes, absolutely. When you first learn to run energy, you will probably amaze your friends with your new found skill. With regular practice, your strength will continue to develop even further. Running the energy is a skill that requires mental and physical concentration. Like an athlete who uses various muscles, you will get stronger. I would estimate that after 100 hours of running energy, your strength will have doubled or possibly tripled.

What if I do not practice for a long time? Will I lose my ability?

When you walk down the street, you don't have to worry about falling off the sidewalk. When you answer the phone, you don't worry that you will forget how to speak. Learning to run energy and do Quantum-Touch is far easier than learning to walk or to talk. Once you have learned the basic skills, they are yours for life. Within hours of picking up this book, you will be able to do profound healing work.

If you have not been running the energy for a while, as in months or years, you may want to spend five or ten minutes building up the energy before you give a session. Another option is to build the energy during the session. Simply practice running the energy while you are giving a session.

Should you run the energy when you are by yourself?

It is a great idea to run the energy whenever you think of it. I usually run the energy for about five minutes before I get out of bed in the morning and another five minutes before I go to sleep. Then throughout the day, from time to time, I will run the energy.

I worry that I am never doing it well enough. What can I do to be sure that I'm running the energy correctly?

This fear of inadequacy is often something that has been learned in other arenas of one's life, like taking a college entrance examination or a test to get a driver's license, but it does not apply to Quantum-Touch.

When you are eating at your favorite restaurant, you don't worry that you will forget how to swallow or pick up your fork. These abilities are totally natural. If you are feeling your hands, can do a full body sweep and do the breathing techniques, then you are doing it well enough. Now it is just a matter of practice and discovering your gifts. You can't do it wrong. Over time you can learn to do it better and more powerfully.

So far I haven't met anyone who complained that a miracle took six sessions instead of one!

One fear people have is that they don't feel loving or spiritual enough to do great work. I remember on one occasion, I had a session scheduled on a day that I was extremely depressed and upset. The woman I was working on had a severe neck problem. So there I was, just running the energy as well as I could. She was lying on her back on my table and I was sitting on a chair holding her neck. Since I was holding this one position for over forty minutes, I rested my head on the top of the table. Then with a start, I realized that I had fallen asleep during the session. I checked my watch and found I was asleep for over ten minutes, yet my hands were still running energy with tremendous intensity. At the end of the session, the woman I was working on told me that that had been the best session that she had ever received.

I have come to recognize that self-doubt is something that many people feel in other arenas of their lives and bring to Quantum-Touch. For many practitioners, the only thing that finally cures their self-doubt is experience. Seeing how incredibly effective you can be on your friend's neck, back, and other pains will eventually convince you that you are doing fabulous work.

There is no substitute for experience.

Is it important for the person receiving the Quantum-Touch session or for the practitioner to believe that it will help for it to work?

As I wrote in my first book, *Your Healing Hands*, you don't have to believe in the ocean to get wet, but you do have to jump in. The same is true here – you don't need to believe in the Quantum-Touch work in order to strongly experience it. Cynics and skeptics do not intellectually know how to block the energy. Quantum-Touch works, period.

What are the biggest mistakes you see first-time practitioners make that keep them from being effective?

By and large, first-time practitioners are actually quite skilled and effective in this work. But to answer this question, there are three mistakes that beginners often make. The first one is to forget to keep the breathing going. I encourage all the Quantum-Touch instructors to kindly nag their students to keep their breathing going. "Keep breathing" becomes sort of a mantra that is repeated every ten minutes during the practice sessions. "Keep breathing – always keep breathing!"

The second mistake is that beginners often need to learn to relax their hands. It is actually much easier to run the energy when your hands are relaxed. I'll go around the room during a workshop checking everyone's hands to get them to relax. I'll take people's hands and shake them lightly, encouraging them to relax them more. The work of Quantum-Touch is done with energy, and clenched and tight hands are not helpful and may work to block the energy.

The third mistake is to quit working before the session is finished. Whether you are working on a chronic or an acute difficulty, beginners tend to want to stop before the healing is completed. The rule of thumb is that when you think you are finished running energy into an area that needs it, it is a good idea to spend at least a few extra minutes working on that area. The two reasons for this are as follows:

You may find that the resonance (as noted by the amount of sensation in your hands) is ready to increase again if you stay in one place longer. New practitioners are often inexperienced at judging how long to run energy into an area.

Running energy for a longer period of time can often help secure the new vibration in the tissue so that their healing tends to last longer.

Quantum-Touch and Personal Energy

Are you using up your own personal energy when you do Quantum-Touch?

Absolutely not. We are using the power of our love and the power of our intent. Based on experience, I'd say that the more of this energy that you use, the more you have. You simply don't run out. When you love someone a great deal, you don't walk around drained and miserable all day whining, "Poor me, I've used up all my love for the day. I have no more to give." Anyway, let's hope you don't. When you love a great deal, you feel like you have far more love to give, and often in all directions. Everyone in your sphere may become a beneficiary of your love – from friends you see to strangers on the street. Quite simply, the more love you feel, the more you have to give. Similarly with intent: the more you use the power of your intention, the more intention you have available.

Do you ever become drained when you do Quantum-Touch sessions?

No, you don't become drained at all. As I have mentioned a number of times, the breathing techniques are an essential part of the work. As long as you keep the breathing up, you will be able to maintain a very high resonance. The other person simply and automatically starts to match your vibration. You are really not giving your energy away; you are holding a field and letting the other person come and match that field, so you don't become drained doing Quantum-Touch. If anything, it is quite the opposite: doing the work seems to cause the practitioner to feel more healed and uplifted. Personally, when I do hours of healing work, it makes me very hungry, and that is one symptom which is easily corrected.

A few practitioners have complained that they felt so energized from doing sessions late at night that they had trouble sleeping. This seems to happen to a small percentage of people using Quantum-Touch, so I'd recommend that they do their sessions earlier in the day. Occasionally, someone doing a session may feel tired afterwards, but this appears to be their reaction to receiving a healing themselves while they were doing the work. Remember, when you are giving a session, you are raising your vibration, which causes healing inside you. Sometimes you may need to sleep afterwards. This however, has nothing to do with having your energy drained out of you.

I find that when I do Quantum-Touch sessions, I often feel more awake after the session than when I began. Why is that?

When you are running the energy and doing the breathing work, you are also benefiting from the energy. There have been a number of times when I felt tired when I was about to give a lecture with demonstrations. As I am giving the short demonstration sessions to the audience, I have consistently found that I become increasingly awake and energized. By the time I have done 20 or 30 demonstration healing sessions at the lecture, I am quite energized and awake. The longer you run the energy, the stronger you seem to get both physically and energetically.

When you run energy, do you find by the end of the day that the energy is not as strong as when you began?

I find quite the opposite. The longer you run energy, the stronger you seem to get. During large lectures where I may be running energy on dozens of people for two hours or more, the later sessions that I give are far stronger than the earlier ones. Sometimes the energy gets so strong that people actually may feel a little jolt as a huge surge of energy moves through them the second they are touched. I may be physically tired from lecturing for two hours and doing so many healing sessions, but the energy is not at all diminished. If anything, it is greatly increased.

Preparation for a Quantum-Touch Session

What should I do to prepare myself to give a session?

If you want to prepare ahead of time, it can be useful to do full body sweeps and see how intensely you can feel the energy throughout your body. While you are doing them, it is also useful to be using any of the breathing techniques to raise up your energy. Most practitioners find that just giving a session will do these things as well.

Is it important to ground myself before giving a session?

For those unfamiliar with the term "grounding," it refers to the practice of centering your energies and often connecting yourself to the earth. In this way people feel more balanced and less vulnerable to picking up unwanted energy. I don't find it necessary to ground myself as long as I do full body sweeps and keep the breathing going. Some people find grounding exercises helpful as they may feel a bit lightheaded from the work. Other people find that the process of running energy itself automatically grounds them.

A few of my students who have told me that they can see energy have been quite surprised when the class finished doing "full body sweeps" because everyone in the room had become grounded.

If you wish to ground yourself in addition to doing full body sweeps, here is an easy approach. Imagine a beam of light coming down into the top of your head, going through your torso, down your legs, into your feet, and into the earth. Sense it going deeply into the earth and linking to the earth. Take a few deep breaths, breathing in the earth energy and feeling yourself grounding. A secret to this approach to grounding is to do it in such a way as to cause yourself to have tactile sensations throughout your body. While you are doing this, start up the 2-6 breathing pattern. Once you have gone through your whole body, extend your body sensations into the earth. This exercise need only take a minute or two to complete. Once you are grounded, take a few minutes and run the energy through your whole body. By now you are quite ready to begin a session.

Is it important for the person you are working on to take off their clothes?

In a Quantum-Touch session, removing a person's clothing is not necessary at all. It can be useful if they take off any heavy clothing, such as jackets or sweaters. I would recommend that people remove anything made of leather during this work. This may sound strange, but the leather blocks the flow of the life-force energy. Synthetic fibers such as polyester diminish the amount of energy flow, so I suggest you wear cotton, wool, or silk.

Using Your Hands in a Quantum-Touch Session

How much pressure do you place in your hands when you run energy?

You really don't need any pressure at all. A light touch works the best. I tell my students this and five minutes later, as I'm walking around the room touching their hands, I find that many of them are holding a good deal of tension in their hands and fingers. At this point, I take hold of their hand and shake it a bit to give them the sense of letting go of the tension. Many people get accustomed to using force in massage, acupressure, shiatsu, rolfing, deep tissue work, and so on. The great irony is that you can unwind and release the tension better in muscles if you use no pressure, or very little. The secret is in using the energy rather than using brute force. In most cases, the use of force is counterproductive.

It is actually easier to run energy when your hands are very relaxed. Since I am not with you to grab your hand and shake it lightly to help release the tension, you might try this simple exercise. Close your hands gently into soft fists, and feel your hands completely relax. Try running energy into your hands. Notice how the energy flows. Now try making tight fists, and try running the energy into your hands. You will probably find that it is much harder to feel the energy when you are straining.

Why is it important to surround areas you are working on with your hands? Why not use just one hand?

Having two points of contact creates a stronger field of vibration between you and the person you are working on. Sandwiching a painful spot between your hands is a excellent way to raise the resonance of the tissue. As I describe in the section about group sessions in chapter 5, when you have four hands or even six working, they can quickly become the dominant resonance. I highly recommend that you always use both hands whenever possible. Furthermore, I suggest that you put your hands on both sides of the problem area to sandwich it between your hands.

I notice that sometimes when you are demonstrating Quantum-Touch, you use your palms, other times you use your thumbs or fingertips. Why do you do this?

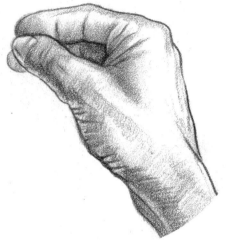

When I want to concentrate the energy into a small area such as the TMJ point (see p. 145) or on the sides of the vertebrae, I will use my fingertips to concentrate the energy. This is a technique that Bob Rasmusson came up with that he called the "tripod." Simply touch your thumb, index finger, and middle finger together and direct the energy out of your fingertips. Focusing the energy in this manner can help you to be more effective when working in very small places.

Using the palms of your hands is recommended for the vast majority of the time. If it is physically awkward or uncomfortable for you to use your palms during a session, use your fingertips or a tripod. Don't let the rules I'm giving you get in the way of putting your hands on someone to do the healing work. Above all, be comfortable when you are doing Quantum-Touch.

I have no sensation in my hands or any part of my body – what should I do?

I have found in my classes that a small percentage of people have trouble feeling sensations. This makes it a bit tougher to learn to do Quantum-Touch, but with time and persistence these people have learned to run energy quite well. A few of the best healers I know have had a difficult time feeling some part of their bodies when they first started out.

The first question to ask yourself is whether or not you have any sensation anywhere in your body that you can feel without touching. Can you feel any part of your body without touching yourself? If you can feel your hands, feet, face, or any other part of your body by bringing your attention there, then you have a starting place and you can build from there.

The Power of Focused Energy

How important is it to be focused during the sessions?

To really boost the power of your sessions, it can make a big difference to try to focus 100 percent on running the energy. Clearly this requires a great deal of effort on the part of the practitioner. When I say "effort," I mean to concentrate on running the energy, concentrate on the breath, and consistently connecting the energy to your breath. Those who have developed a great deal of skill in running energy often speak of completely giving themselves to the process.

If I concentrate 100 percent on running the energy, does that mean I should never talk while giving a session?

Not necessarily. I strongly recommend that you concentrate on having fun when you are doing Quantum-Touch sessions. The work is about love, joy, gratitude, and wonder, not about rigidity or being overly serious. When you are about to drive your car onto a highway and need to accelerate, it may take a lot of gas to get the car up to speed. Once it is up to speed, you can let up on the gas and cruise. Similarly, when you are running energy, it may take a lot of work to bring the vibration up to a "high pitch." Once you have done so, you can keep the breathing going and let the energy continue to do the work.

It is OK to talk with your client from time to time. The important thing is to be sure that you continue using your breathing techniques while you talk. If you make an effort, you can take big breaths while you speak. Be sure to keep asking your client about what they are experiencing, as this can give you valuable information. Continuing with the car analogy, you may want to accelerate in order to pass another car on the road. In Quantum-Touch, at times you may want to do some fire breaths to bring the energy up to a higher vibration. At this point, you would stop talking and focus 100 percent on running the energy.

The Client's Experience of a Quantum-Touch Session

How long does it take for people to know that something is happening when they receive a session?

Often people will notice energy shifts and changes in their pain levels within a few seconds of being touched. During my lectures, I like to give as many three or four minute sessions as I can. I'll ask people to tell me about only one area where they are in pain. If I have a large audience, I'll often bring some of my students or other Quantum-Touch teachers on stage to help out. Typically, about 90 percent of the people receiving these short sessions will report a major shift in symptoms. Many times, people will approach me six months or a year later and tell me that the pain didn't came back, even though the session was rather brief.

I like doing these short sessions because it makes the work believable. People often need to feel the energy for themselves before they are willing to believe in it or use it.

What do people usually feel when they receive a Quantum-Touch session?

People are all unique and will experience the energy in their own fashion. Some people will not feel the energy at all. Many will experience the energy as hot, cold, or tingling sensations. It is important to understand that all sensations that a person experiences from the work – from the most minor to the most intense – are all excellent signals that the session is working. The most common sensation that people feel is that of heat. The heat can be mild and slightly warming all the way to burning and painful. If a light touch is capable of bringing up strong physical pain, however uncomfortable it may be for the client in the short run, it is a very positive sign that you are making wonderful progress in the healing. I remember with one student who worked on me during a class, it didn't just feel hot on my lower back where he was working, it actually felt quite sunburned.

Is it the temperature of your hand people are responding to when they say they are feeling hot or cold sensations?

This does not seem to be the case. Recently I worked on a man who felt a burning heat when I was working on his back. I let him touch my fingers and to his great surprise, he found that my fingers were actually quite cold. When I touched his back again, there was the same burning sensation as before. A little later, he felt the sensation as cool around his hips. It is a bit unusual for a person to feel both heat and coolness from the energy, but it does happen.

On another occasion, I was working on a man who had problems with his arm. This fellow was certain that the burning heat he felt was due to my body heat. To prove to himself that it was a purely physical sensation, he put on a down coat, which would insulate any heat coming from my hands. I had a good laugh because he just about jumped out of his chair when he felt the same burning sensation as before, right through his coat.

The sensation of heat is probably the most common thing that people report from Quantum-Touch sessions. Other common sensations that people experience during sessions include feeling cold, tingling or vibration, and pain.

Is it ever painful to receive the energy?

Yes, occasionally it is. Sometimes people feel a painful reaction when they are receiving energy. This pain doesn't usually last very long. I don't like seeing people in pain, but I always get excited when this happens since it has consistently been a strong indication that a major healing is taking place. The key here is to continue doing the session at least until the pain has gone away.

A few years ago, my friend Dan asked me if I would work on his 13-year-old son who had broken his knee and was still limping after the cast was removed. When I first started running energy into his knee, he protested, "Ouch, you're hurting me. It feels like my knee is killing me." I told him to breathe deeply and that the sensations would not last long. About two minutes later he protests, "Now my knee is on fire. What are you doing to me?" I explained that this was all part of the healing process. Another couple of minutes passed and he said that now his knee felt all "pins and needles," and two minutes after that, he said that his knee felt all warm and wonderful. After about twelve minutes his knee was fine and he didn't limp again.

Do you ever get clues about other places that need healing energy other than those places that specifically hurt?

There are two ways of doing this. The first way involves the use of anatomical knowledge and logic. Guidelines about this can be found in various chapters of this book. The second way involves letting the body tell you exactly where the energy is needed, and in my opinion, the second way is far more profound. Often when you run energy into one place for a period of time, the person's body will prioritize the use of the energy as it sees fit. As is the case of all healing, the entire process is quite automatic. The only logic and reason behind this is the magnificence of the body's own innate intelligence.

If you were working on someone's lower back pain for example, they may report back to you that they are now feeling a sensation or even a pain somewhere else, perhaps higher up in the back or possibly in the neck, knee, or wherever. I like to ask clients to tell me if they are feeling the energy going to some place other than where I am working. As their body intelligence directs the life-force to specific areas of their body, the person receiving the session will likely get corresponding sensations that they can report.

When a person tells you that they are experiencing energy going to some other part of their body, I suggest that you make a mental note of it. As soon as you are finished running energy into the area where you are working, you simply bring your hands to the area that now feels the new sensation or pain and work on that area as well. This is what I call "chasing the pain." In many cases, you will simply chase the pain from one place to another until it is gone.

On one occasion, I was demonstrating Quantum-Touch on an acupuncturist who had a number of burns on the back of her hand. When I ran the energy into her hand, I asked her to describe what she was feeling. She told me that all the energy was going into her elbow. When I inquired why her elbow needed energy, she explained that she had broken it two years ago and that it had never healed properly. At that point, I discontinued working on her hand and started working on her elbow. The energy surged into her elbow for about five minutes. When the energy had shifted and became less intense, I asked her how her elbow was feeling. She was amazed that all the pain and discomfort in her elbow was gone.

It is common for beginning students to discover that when they are working on a lower back condition, at some point in the session the client will report that they are having energy rushes into their neck. Since the neck and lower back reflex each other, the body is saying that it is important to work on both areas. Similarly, when working on a repetitive stress injury on the wrist, people often report feeling energy going into their elbow, shoulder, neck, head, or back. These points are most likely involved in the condition and will show up through this process of secondary sensations.

Does the energy ever heal conditions other than what you think you are working on?

This often happens. Since the energy will go where "it wants," all sorts of surprise healings occur. The most common are the people with headaches who discover that their sinus pain disappeared as well. It works the other way too. People complaining of sinus pain often report that their headaches have disappeared.

On one occasion during one of my classes, two students were working on a woman who had sharp sinus pains. When the session was over, the woman said that she still had painful sinuses. I explained that it is not a perfect system and to give it time. The next morning she called me to say that her sinuses still hurt. I told her that this happens occasionally. She went on to say that her eyesight which has always been 20/200 in her right eye had suddenly changed, and it was now 20/25, but her sinuses still hurt! She was overjoyed.

Incidentally, her eyesight did not stabilize at 20/25, but has been fluctuating since that time. As she continues to run energy into her eyes it is gradually improving.

If the energy automatically travels to the places that need it, why is it important to try to put your hands directly on those parts of the body that are most problematic?

If you had an unlimited amount of time, it truly wouldn't matter. Given time constraints, it is just a whole lot faster and more efficient to go to those specific places that require the healing. You could fill the swimming pool by turning on a hose in your garden, but it would be a lot easier to put the hose directly into the pool.

Quantum-Touch and the Emotions

How does Quantum-Touch affect the emotions of the person I'm working on?

The emotions of the client will usually become much more balanced and harmonious. The energy does not differentiate between physical and emotional problems. It goes where it is needed and does what is needed for the person. I remember on one occasion I came to visit a friend to do some work. He warned me when I came in the door, "I need to warn you that I'm feeling very cranky today." I asked him, "Where in your body are you feeling cranky?" He said, "That's a very interesting question — I'm feeling it in my upper chest, throat, and back of my neck." I told him to sit down and I would see what I could do. I just ran energy for about six or eight minutes into those places. To his amazement, when I was done, his crankiness had lifted. "What did you do to me?" he asked. "Oh", I said, "I just gave you an attitude adjustment."

The purpose of the Quantum-Touch sessions is not to heal the emotional problems of your client, but rather to help them find a place of greater emotional balance and of feeling centered so that they can more effectively and responsibly work with and process their own emotions. I know of one psychotherapist who uses Quantum-Touch to great advantage with her clients. She asks the client in what part of the body that the emotions are being felt. Then with the permission of the client she places her hands on those places and runs the energy. She is extremely careful to make sure that there is no sexual innuendo or implications through this touch. The result is that her clients move into a place where they can more effectively deal with their emotions.

Emotional issues that are unresolved can block the healing vibrations or cause the disease state to return. This work does not relieve the patients from having to do their personal emotional and psychological transformational healing. If Quantum-Touch were able to take the place of emotional processing and healthy expression of emotions, I would consider it a hindrance. I believe that learning to be emotionally honest with ourselves and to feel and release our emotions is a primary skill. Anything that interferes with that fundamental part of our growth would be counterproductive. Fortunately, Quantum-Touch only assists people to be in a more balanced place, where they can then do the expressing, forgiving, and releasing necessary for their growth.

How will Quantum-Touch affect my emotions when I use it?

Each time that a practitioner of Quantum-Touch is running energy – whether by him or herself in practice doing full body sweeps or working on a client – the practitioner is raising their own vibration and receiving some benefit from the energy. Beyond this mild healing from just running the energy, the act of giving has been known to work wonders for the emotional state of the practitioner. I have experienced it myself and have been told by numerous students of Quantum-Touch how giving a session lifted their emotions.

Ending a Quantum-Touch Session

Do the sensations in your hands change when it is time for the session to end?

I have found this to be the case. When the client has had all the energy that they can handle, their body will simply not accept any more, and you may feel the tingling or other sensations in your hands will slow down or stop. In many cases, over time, you may feel their body slowly matching the energy vibration of your hands. When the vibrations become the same, you may no longer be able to feel any sensation whatsoever as long as you are touching them. It's funny, but everyone doing Quantum-Touch work seems to think, "I must not be running the energy because I feel nothing in my hands." Then when you take your hands away from your friend, you will feel your hands buzzing like crazy. Place your hands back on the other person again, and you'll feel nothing. This is normal. It is a sign that the process is completed for now.

I have a secret technique that I use. I like to ask the person how they are feeling. If they are still in pain, I tend to feel that the session is not over. I can't always get to this point however. With practice, you will get a sense of how far a person is willing to shift their vibration in any given session.

The person I was working on wanted me to stop after ten minutes and told me that she felt that that was all the energy that her body could take. Is this true?

Once in a while, the energy feels uncomfortable to the person who is receiving it, as their reaction to the healing is quite intense. This is understandable. If you stop at this time, be aware that the session is not over and you may leave the person in that uncomfortable state. If a person is having this sort of strong reaction to the healing, I recommend that you gently encourage them to continue with the session. Over time, as the energy balances out, the reaction should feel diminished to both you and your client or friend. Stopping when the energy is intense like that would be premature.

How do you determine how many sessions a person will need?

There are no hard and fast rules about how many sessions a person will need. If a person has had a long chronic condition, it often takes longer to help than one that is acute or more recent. The rule of thumb is to continue working on a client as long as they need help. I would let the client decide how often they need to come in. For certain conditions they may want a session two or three times a week or perhaps even every day for a few days. It all depends. There would be no harm in scheduling a series of sessions for a chronic back condition. In the long run, it is important for me to see that I am making progress.

After a Session

What can your client do after a session to improve their own healing?

After the session is over, if the person receiving it is able to continue to run the energy through the parts of their body you worked on, they can intensify and prolong the healing effects.

Is there something you should do for your client or friend after a session is completed?

I suggest that you give them a glass of water to drink. As a result of the session, toxins may be released and drinking water can help wash them away. I think it is a wonderful idea to charge a glass of water by running energy into it for them to drink. (see p. 196) When the session is over, your hands are still running energy at a very high vibration. You can probably charge an eight ounce glass of water quite powerfully in about three to five minutes.

Can Quantum-Touch be Harmful?

Can you ever harm someone by running too much energy into them?

To the best of my knowledge, this has never happened. You really can't give someone too much energy. If a part of the body gets more energy than it needs, it sends the overflow of energy to some other part of the body that needs it more. The receiver will feel sensations going to some other place, which can be useful information. When I visited with Dr. Norman Shealy and taught him to run the energy, this question came up. From his perspective, you cannot harm the person because this energy is only balancing. When balance has been obtained, the energy will cease to flow or it will just pass on through.

Is there any danger in doing Quantum-Touch?

Quantum-Touch to the best of my knowledge is not dangerous. I have seen it work wonders on newborn babies, animals, and the elderly. In over twenty years, I have not seen anything deleterious. As I said before, if you give a person more energy than they can use, their body will simply not absorb it.

I can think of one case where I would be afraid to give a person a Quantum-Touch session. A few years ago, I met a man who had had liver transplant surgery and was taking medication to suppress his immune system from rejecting his new liver. My concern was that giving him energy might cause his immune system to function more efficiently and thus he could be in danger of liver failure. Since I don't know this to be the case, I would err on the side of caution.

Can people use these techniques to harm others?

Theoretically yes, but I don't know anyone who has tried. The problem with trying to use the energy in a negative way is that it so quickly comes back to haunt the perpetrator. For whatever reasons, the world seems to be set up in such a way that you tend to rapidly get what you are giving out. Aside from this, consciously harming other people is a guaranteed way to diminish one's self-esteem. To anyone tempted to vent their hatred in this manner, I could only suggest that he or she find some healthy ways to release their anger, which can be incredibly empowering.

Quantum-Touch and Other Modalities

Do you have any suggestions for using Quantum-Touch in conjunction with other hands-on healing techniques?

Oh, yes. To the best of my knowledge, Quantum-Touch can be used to work with or enhance the power of any other form of hands-on healing modality. I consider it to be a transparent therapy because it is so easily used with other forms of practice. If you are using Reiki, simply do Quantum-Touch during your Reiki sessions. For practitioners of shiatsu or acupressure, just run the energy out of your thumbs or fingers as you normally practice your work. Massage practitioners have found that it takes a good deal of concentration to be able to run the energy during the session. With some practice, they can become skilled at doing this. I am told that clients report that after a Quantum-Touch massage session, they feel as if they are glowing. Chiropractors have found that they can use Quantum-Touch in place of most "high speed" adjustments. Cranial sacral therapists have told me that this work has transformed their practice. The list just goes on and on. Essentially, Quantum-Touch can add to the effectiveness of many other techniques.

Can Anybody Learn to Do Quantum-Touch?

Can people with handicaps or blind or deaf people learn to do Quantum-Touch work?

Oh, yes. Running energy is dependent on intention, attention, and breathing. A person who does not have the distractions of sight or sound may hold their focus as well, and potentially do even better than their seeing or hearing counterparts.

Can children learn to do Quantum-Touch?

Absolutely. Children usually have no problem learning to do this work. If they have a desire to do healing work, they can be as effective as adults. It is not uncommon for children to take my class, and much to the delight of their parents, they do wonderful healing work.

In one class I taught, a woman brought her 11-year-old son Zack to class. Zack had a wonderful time discovering that he could do healing work every bit as well as the adults, and he was able to help his mom as she worked on his numerous skating injuries and postural misalignments. The love he and his mother were sharing was one of the most beautiful things that I had ever seen.

On the way back home, Zack said, "You know, I was secretly wishing that I had super-human powers, and now I feel like I do." The next day at school, Zack told his best friend that he had learned to heal people. His friend said, "Heal me." Zack asked his friend where he hurt. The friend replied that he didn't hurt anywhere. Zack told him, "I can't help you unless you are in pain." With that, Zack's friend slammed his own hand down onto the table as hard as he could. The hand was swelling and changing color. Zack calmly picked up the hand and started running energy into it. A few minutes later, Zack's friend said, "Wow, that's so cool." Then the two of them ran off to play.

Do you have to be intuitive when you do this sort of work?

Being intuitive is in no way a prerequisite for being successful when you do Quantum-Touch. While some people seem to naturally have an automatic sense of knowing exactly where to place their hands, I have found that worlds of good can be accomplished by using the "where does it hurt?" technique. The majority of great results that I have seen have employed this "low tech" way of knowing.

How different are Quantum-Touch practitioners from one to another?

Just as every flower is unique and beautiful, each practitioner seems to have a unique and beautiful energy. Not everyone's energies are equal. Some practitioners seem to do well with broken bones, others may do well with tumors. I find that I do especially well with injuries, inflammation, structural alignment, and pain reduction. Other healers seem to have gifts in other areas. I believe that one day we will have ways of determining where a person's expertise may be when working with Quantum-Touch. Beyond this, I think at some point in the future, we will find that various people will be able to specialize in areas such as trauma care, heart disease, cancer, and so forth.

Could you give me a few pointers about doing a Quantum-Touch session?

- Always keep your breathing techniques going.

- Always keep your breath connected to your sensations while running the energy. (This quickly becomes a habit and second nature to practitioners.)

- Stay focused to keep the energy as strong as you can.

- Pay close attention to what you are feeling in your hands and use that information appropriately.

I'm still confused. How can I be doing Quantum-Touch work and not be a healer?

Our language can be so lacking in some areas. The person doing the Quantum-Touch work is not really a "healer," although he or she is clearly doing healing. When we do Quantum-Touch work, we are creating a field of energy with our hands. With that energy, we create a vibrational environment so the person getting worked on can heal themselves. It is my belief that we are really not using up our own energy when we work on someone else, but rather, we are using the energy of the universe to hold this field of energy in their proximity. Their body understands this field of energy, and through the power of resonance and entrainment, their cells gradually match the vibration of your hands. Somehow in this process, their "body intelligence" and "spiritual intelligence" use this new vibration to cause healing as appropriate to the needs of the recipient.

In the same way that no one can eat for you or laugh for you, no one can heal for you. No matter how much healing work you receive from other people, keep in mind that it is your body and only your body that is doing the healing. Simply stated, your body heals itself. In my opinion, anyone who claims that they can heal you does not understand the mechanism of healing.

The person who is doing the "healing" work is there to create the environment for healing to take place, no more and no less. So when I tell people that my profession is that of a healer, I am using the common jargon. Few people would understand me if I said that I hold a resonance so people can harmonically entrain to my vibration to heal themselves.

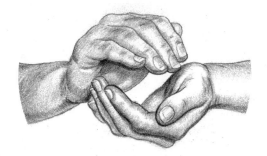

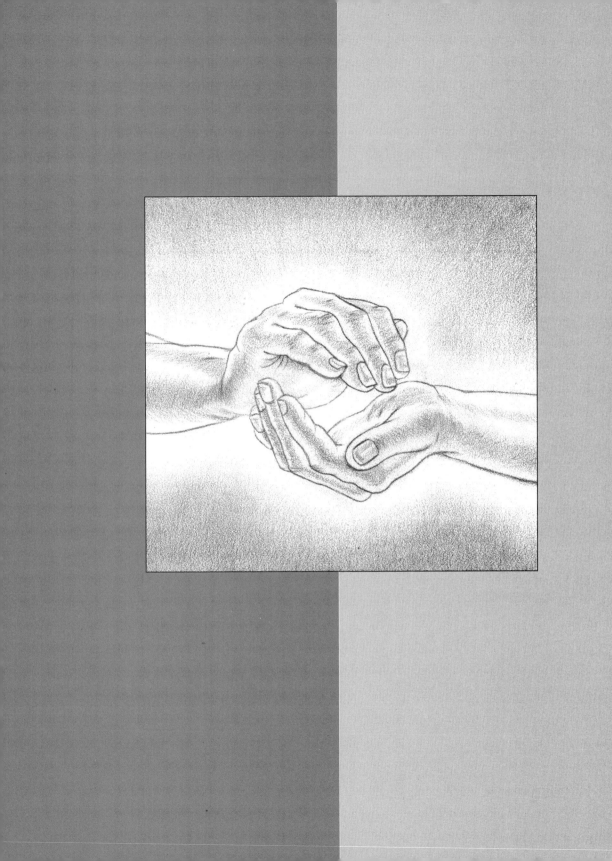

Chapter 5

Intermediate Techniques

The life-force is an energy that surrounds and penetrates all living things. Perhaps the same can be said of love. The intimate connection between the life-force and our love is one of the great and persisting mysteries.

If you have been able to do the energy and breathing exercises outlined in chapter 3, you have already learned the basic skills you need to be an unusually powerful healing practitioner. The easiest way you will know this to be true is by doing the work on people who are in pain.

At this point, you are ready to begin learning the intermediate techniques. These skills will further empower the basic techniques, but are not a substitute for them. I strongly suggest that you keep practicing the introductory techniques also – you can never practice them too much. The intermediate techniques I will be sharing with you are optional, in the sense that some practitioners will gravitate to and embrace certain of these techniques and not others. I suggest that you find the techniques that you enjoy most and that work best for you.

Resonance Factors

When I teach people to run energy, I want them to see how easy it is to powerfully effect changes. If you have practiced the techniques in chapter 3, you will have discovered this for yourself. Now is a great time to consider what I call "resonance factors" in running the energy. These resonance factors are things you can do to lift your resonance and improve upon the quality and the power of your healing work. I like to present these factors at this time because they build on what you have already learned, and because they can make your healing sessions even more powerful.

Take your time to think about and truly work with these resonance factors as they will greatly enhance your healing sessions.

1. **Run the energy —** The full body sweeps and other body-oriented techniques that intensify your own physical body sensation and bring it out your hands are an essential component of Quantum-Touch. The more sensation you are able to generate in your body through your intention and attention, the more effective your work will be.

2. **Use the breathing techniques** — Like the bellows heating a blacksmith's fire, breathing is an essential component in raising the resonance of your healing work. Running the energy by itself is valuable, but combining it with the breathing is many times more powerful than doing just one or the other. Generally speaking, the larger the volume of air that you are moving, the more effective your work will be. Remember to always breathe throughout your sessions. This not only raises your vibration for healing, but it is simultaneously the way you will protect yourself from picking up the other person's energy from a session and becoming depleted. Breathe big breaths, the more air the better, as long as you do not become dizzy.

3. **Connect your breath with the energy** — More important than simply doing the breathing or running the energy, is connecting the two together. With practice, the breathing and your sensations will become completely linked. When your breath and the sensations in your hands are fully connected, you will be able to feel how each breath you are taking is affecting and often increasing the sensations in your hands. It is at this point that you are truly doing the work well. Like blowing on hot embers to make them brighter, the more air you move, the more powerful your energy tends to be.

4. **Remember your intention** — Your intention to heal is an important aspect of the work. For most people, this desire to assist another in their healing is a natural and almost instinctive response. When we see someone in pain, we feel a desire to help. This reaction and desire to help is all that is required.

   It may surprise you, but you can be quite angry, depressed, grieving, or even outraged, and still do a wonderful job of "healing." The very process of doing Quantum-Touch will in most cases lift your emotions. Your simple intention to help is sufficient to do the work very well. When I speak of "having the intention to heal," some people begin to doubt themselves and their intentions. The truth is, their desire to heal was already evident in the fact that they attended my workshop, or are taking the time to read this book. You don't have to wait till you are "perfect" or in some holy or enlightened state to help. Furthermore, it is important to realize that your intention actually transcends your current emotional state. That is, your desire to heal matters far more than the particular emotions you may be feeling at any given moment.

5. **Choose to feel love and gratitude** — As you have seen, just running energy through your body and connecting it to the breathing techniques can cause you to have tremendous healing power. I described earlier how I believe that it is our nature to love and how the simple act of watching a child play can cause that child to feel loved, since the act of attention is a form of loving. We do not have to "try" to be loving during a session because that is our nature. Dogs do not have to try to be "doglike," and trees do not have to try to act more "treelike." Humans are naturally loving creatures, and in Quantum-Touch, we do not have to make any special effort to be so. This is why just running the energy can cause such profound and magnificent results.

    Having said that, I will tell you that you can make the work even better for yourself and the person you are working on by consciously choosing to enter states of love and or gratitude. Whatever you do, don't force yourself to try to feel something that you are not. If you are not feeling loving or grateful, don't feel guilty that you are doing a bad session (because you are not). But if you are able, consciously call forth your own feelings of love and gratitude. Let yourself fully enjoy and feel the tactile sensations in your body that love or gratitude will cause you to feel. The gratitude or love can be about anything in your life. The key here is raising your vibration. I think that you will be very happy with the results. Love and gratitude are the opposite of self-pity and self-importance, which are resonance factors that you would do best to avoid. Consciously placing yourself in a state of gratitude can lift your resonance and profoundly improve your work.

6. **Hold a positive expectation** — Holding an honest expectation that the body not only can heal, but has the wisdom to do so, can lift and improve your resonance. The trick to expectation is to always be completely honest about where you are and to expect the best based on your level of experience and confidence. A great starting place is to say to yourself, "I don't know if it is possible to heal this or not, but I'm willing to see what happens, and I know that the body has a blueprint of wholeness that it can access." You don't have to know how that is possible, just be open to the fact that that is true. As you do so, keep in mind that the body has a wisdom and an ability to heal itself that far surpasses human comprehension. Holding the belief that it is possible that miracles might happen opens windows of possibility. As intention and attention are needed to run the energy, expectation is a potent and valuable factor in raising your vibration. Many of the greatest healers I have known have held a steadfast knowledge and expectation that incredible healings happen quite often and approach their sessions with a joyous sense of positive expectation.

7. **Ask for help** — For those who operate with a spiritual belief system, it can only make things better if you ask for help from a higher power, however you perceive it. Sincerely asking for help is a great thing to do. Here is a big tip: When you do ask for help, feel the tactile sensations of the help you are receiving.

8. **Give your All** — The value of this cannot be overstated. When you give a session, put yourself into it 100 percent, and the results will be greatly improved. Giving your all can mean letting go of any other thoughts, concentrating on your breathing and linking the sensations in your hands, getting out of the way, and even losing track of time and space. Sometimes when you give your all, you feel as if you disappeared in the process – that is, you seem to get out of the way and let the energy do its work. Giving your all can be felt as working as hard as you can, in as a relaxed a state as you can. There need be no tension in your body, your hands, or for that matter, your mind.

9. **Let go of attachment to outcome** — As you recall, I spoke about how the definition of a great healer is someone who was very sick and got well quickly. If you think about this, it becomes clear that the "healer" is truly a healing facilitator. When you do Quantum-Touch, you are really not healing anyone. What you are doing is raising a field of vibration to allow the vibration of their body to be lifted through the power of resonance and entràinment. When you do Quantum-Touch, it is not your responsibility that the person you are working on actually be healed, since you cannot actually heal anyone other than yourself. It is, however, your responsibility to hold the vibration as high as you can for as long as necessary in order to do the best job you can.

There have been times when, despite my best effort, there was no obvious benefit. Just as I truly cannot take the credit for my clients becoming well, I cannot take the blame for them not becoming well. How someone responds to this work is based upon their own ability to receive the healing energy and to hold that vibration. We cannot always judge the effectiveness of what we are doing at the time we are doing it. The job of the healer is to hold the highest vibration they can – period. Sometimes there are factors that keep healing from working at any particular time. Your energy may not be the specific energy they need at this time.

Sometimes, a person may not be ready to be healed: there may be some emotional lessons they need to learn or other factors. Some of these factors may be understood, and others may be beyond our comprehension. The point is that we need not judge ourselves as good or bad or be tied to the outcome of a session. You can hope for the best and even expect the best, but it helps in setting your own resonance to realize that, ultimately, their healing is not your responsibility. You are merely acting as a catalyst to allow your clients to heal themselves.

10. **Trust** — Trusting yourself can have a wonderful effect in keeping your resonance high. This trust has a number of faces: You can trust that your love is good enough, and that your ability to raise your resonance is good enough. You can trust that whatever happens during a session, whether it is an intense emotional release or some sort of dramatic physical release, it is for the best. Finally, you can simply trust the process – whatever it looks like. If symptoms appear to be getting worse, you can maintain an attitude of calm and continue to run the energy with reassuring hands until the pain has run its course.

Take time and consciously apply the resonance factors as you continue to give Quantum-Touch sessions. This may take a bit of effort, but the results are well worth it. The resonance factors can be so much more than a list that you read quickly through. *Give yourself some time to let yourself work with each of the factors and notice how they impact the sensations in your hands.* Make the resonance factors as real as you can and you will see a big improvement in your healing work.

Intermediate Exercises for Running Energy

Creating a Vortex of Energy

Energy does not move in straight lines. From electrons to planets to entire galaxies, everything is in motion, spinning. In terms of mundane physics, a spiraling football or spinning Frisbee cuts through the air more efficiently due to its rotation. Bullets spiral out of a gun, and their spinning motion helps them to go straighter with better penetration. When you get the energy spinning, you are raising both the vibration and the potential for the energy to penetrate.

When you run the energy through your body doing full body sweeps, try spinning it, clockwise or counter-clockwise throughout your entire body. (The direction does not matter.) As you sit or stand, feel the sensation of the energy spinning up your legs, spinning through your torso, into your head, and down your arms and into your hands. When the energy is in your hands, spin it in your palms.

Try vortexing the energy through and around your body at the same time. Speed up the rate of spin by using your intent, and see how much you can feel it.

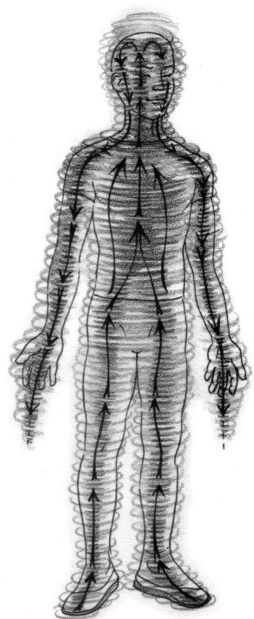

This technique requires a good deal of practice, but it is well worth the time you spend developing your skill. With patience you will be able to feel a great deal of energy spinning powerfully throughout your body any time you choose. Remember, the key here is to use your imagination and intention to cause yourself to feel tactile sensation. The more sensation you feel, the more effective it will be. Simply imagining the energy does not do nearly as much as bringing tactile sensation to the work.

Working with Chakras and Colors

Before I met Rosalyn Bruyere, a highly respected healer, I was told that she could see energy. Despite her excellent reputation, I had become skeptical of anyone who claimed that they could see energy, and I had developed a little test to find out if they were for real. Up to this point, everyone had failed my test. My test consisted of running energy as strongly as I could out of one hand and then casually asking the person to tell me what he or she saw. So when I had the opportunity, I built up a very strong charge in my hand and asked Rosalyn to take a look at the energy in my hand. Rosalyn looked me in the eyes and asked me, "Why are you running all that energy through your hand?" I told her that I wanted to know if she could really see energy. She laughed and said, "I see energy quite clearly, thank you." I got the message.

Rosalyn later went on to explain in her class that when you place your attention into your energy centers known as chakra, the energy coming out your hands takes on the color of the chakra of your attention. Again I tested this out. "What color do you see in my hands now?" I asked, as I held my attention on my third chakra. Without hesitation she said, "Yellow." Two seconds later I asked again as I held my attention in my fifth chakra, "What color do you see now?" Just as quickly she said, "Blue." "OK, what color do you see now?" She said, "Green." I could see that she was becoming bored with the game, but I confirmed, that first, she could truly see energy, and second, that focusing attention on the chakras changes the vibration and color of the energy coming from your hands.

Running the energy through an individual chakra can increase the vibration that you are putting out through your hands. Rather than trying to be psychically or intellectually brilliant in order to figure out exactly which color any part of the body needs, you can put out an entire rainbow spectrum of colors and let the body decide which color it needs and thus choose to draw from. It is what I like to think of as the "multivitamin" approach to healing. Just throw in all the colors and let the body decide on what it needs. Since plants do not do well with a single frequency of light, it seems reasonable that the body does not do well with a single frequency of energy. With both plants and people, I believe that a full spectrum is in order.

Full-Spectrum Chakra Technique

I learned a variation of this technique from a meditation given by a spiritual teacher named Lazaris for working with the chakras and have adapted it for purposes of healing.

First Chakra

Place all your attention in the base of your spine (the end of the tailbone and the area of the perineum between the genitals and the anus) and feel a ball of red light there. The red is a brilliant fire engine red. The tactile sensation is far more important than the visualization. The visualization is primarily used to assist you in bringing about body sensation. Use the 2-6 breathing technique, and on the six-count exhalation, hold your attention in the area of the first chakra.

Once you have tactile sensation in the area of the first chakra, begin spinning the "ball of light" either clockwise or counterclockwise – whichever feels comfortable is fine. The important thing is that your intention is causing increased sensation. Since energy follows thought, the greater your intention and attention, the greater the sensation will become.

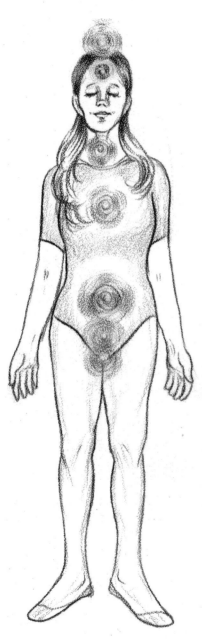

Take a few minutes to see how strongly you can bring sensation to your first chakra.

Second Chakra

Place all your attention to the area of and just behind your genitals. Feel a ball of brilliant orange light, the color like an orange, but glowing. Use the 2-6 breath to send energy into the chakra and spin the ball in whatever direction feels most comfortable. It does not matter if it is in the same direction as the first chakra. Spend a few minutes bringing as much sensation as you can to the second chakra.

Third Chakra

The third chakra is in the area of the solar plexus, above and below your belly button, about the size of your outstretched hand. Feel a ball of brilliant sunny yellow light in your belly, and feel it spin in a comfortable direction. Spend a few minutes bringing as much sensation as you can, and use the 2-6 breath to bring more sensation to this area.

Fourth Chakra

Place your attention in the area of your heart, and feel a ball of brilliant emerald green light about the size of your fist. Get it spinning in whatever direction is comfortable, and use the 2-6 breath to bring more sensation to the area. Spend a few minutes to bring as much sensation to this area as possible.

Fifth Chakra

In the area of your throat, feel a small but intense ball of sapphire sky blue light. Get the ball spinning in whichever direction you find to be comfortable, and again use the 2-6 breath in order to bring more sensation into this chakra. As before, spend a few minutes bringing as much sensation into this area as you can.

Sixth Chakra

In the area above the brow in the center of your forehead is the location of the sixth chakra, sometimes referred to as the third eye. Feel a small glowing ball of indigo light (the color of deep amethyst – a reddish purple) and get it spinning in whichever direction that you find to be comfortable. Use the 2-6 breath to increase intensity of the sensation as you focus on this area for a few minutes.

Seventh Chakra

In the area of the crown of your head, feel a ball of intense violet light. Feel it spinning in the direction of your comfort, using the 2-6 breath to bring more sensation and energy to that area. Spend a few minutes increasing the sensation.

Full Spectrum, One Chakra at a Time

Try running the energy into a person one chakra at a time. Focus on the first chakra and take a few breaths, just spinning that chakra and running the energy out of your hands. Continue this process with each of the other chakras. Be sure to use all seven chakras in this approach so the body can pick and choose the energies it wants to use for its healing process.

In a recent class, one of my students was running the energy through each chakra into his friend. When he got to the sixth chakra, his friend said that she felt as if she were floating. Without saying anything, he tried running the energy again through different chakras into her. Again, each time that he ran energy into her from his sixth chakra, she felt as if she were floating.

The Full Spectrum, All Chakras

Imagine a colored ball of light glowing and spinning at each chakra, but this time work to keep all seven chakras spinning at once. Start at the first, go to the second, third, and so on, but check as you go to make sure that they are all still spinning. As you work your way up to the seventh chakra, give a nudge to any chakras that are not spinning. By the end of this exercise, you should be able to feel all seven chakras spinning at once. When you spin all the colors together, you get a white light. Continue using the 2-6 breath to increase the sensation and power of this exercise.

As a way to facilitate you in doing this, imagine that you have a hand crank, and by turning it, you can get all seven of the chakras spinning at once. Continue using the 2-6 breath as you get them spinning.

Repeat the exercise, except this time, as you get each chakra spinning, imagine that you can hear them spin. The faster they spin, the higher the frequency of the sound. This time get all seven chakras spinning one by one, and hear each of them emitting a sound that gets higher and higher as they go faster. Use your imagination and see if you can feel sparks of light shooting off the chakras as they spin. Continue using the 2-6 breath to increase the power and sensation of this exercise.

It can work wonderfully to get your chakras spinning before you begin a session. Occasionally during the session, you may wish to give them a spin.

Toning

Toning is an extremely powerful way of increasing the impact of your healing sessions. For many people, this becomes their favorite way to run the energy. Toning involves singing a tone out loud or in your mind. When you are doing Quantum-Touch work, you can amplify the intensity of the work by toning mentally or out loud. Since toning out loud may seem strange or socially out of place to many people and may even scare others, it is good to know that toning mentally can work just as well as doing it out loud.

Try closing your hand lightly and start running energy into your hand. Once you get a strong feeling of the energy, try singing a tone out loud. Pay close attention and notice how the energy in your hands has shifted. Now try toning different notes. You can sing a series of higher notes and see which one has the strongest vibration in your hands.

Once you get accustomed to toning out loud, try doing it silently. Mentally tone various notes and pay close attention to the sensations in your hands. Most people will notice that certain mental tones will cause more sensation and certain other tones will produce less sensation.

When you are doing a Quantum-Touch session, simply find the tones (whether out loud or mentally) that cause the greatest sensation in your hands and tone them while running the energy. You can fine-tune the tones by exploring the various vowel sounds to find which one or ones have the greatest resonant qualities.

The problem with toning out loud during a session is that you often slow down your breathing as you are slowly exhaling. When you slow down the breathing, you tend to lower your vibration and become susceptible to picking up energy from the person you are working on. The solution to this problem is to use the "breathy tone" technique.

Breathy Tone Technique

While you are toning, be sure to exhale all of your air to the count of four or six. This produces a rather breathy tone. If you try whispering loudly, you can get a sense of the feel of the breathy tone. It may not sound as nice, but it will keep your energy high so you will be more effective and well protected during your sessions. When you do the toning, it is vital to keep the breathing going just as strongly as when you are not doing the toning. The breathing keeps you from matching the vibration of the person you are working on. Exhaling a great deal of air while you are simultaneously singing the tone will do this.

Having the Client Raise Their Own Vibration

Another way to raise the vibration of a session is for the person who is being worked on to help out. The easiest way to do this is to ask the client to put all of his or her attention to wherever they are being touched. Instruct the client to pay close attention and to feel as much sensation under your hands or in any other part of their body as they can. The second thing to do is to have the client breathe deeply, as if they were breathing directly into the places that you are touching. That is, they should feel as if the breath is coming through the area of contact. The third thing is that the client should report back to you any changes in their sensation in the area you are working or in any other part of their body. You can have them doing a 1-4 breath or a 2-6 breath. Use the 1-4 if they are experiencing pain and the 2-6 or circular breathing during the rest of the session.

By placing their attention in the area being touched, they are bringing their own consciousness to that spot. When they are bringing the power of their breath to the area, they are further raising the vibration, and you will feel increased sensations in your hands. Another way of doing this is to ask your client to match your breathing pattern so your breathing is synchronized. This can be quite dramatic, and the results will speak for themselves.

Stacking Hands and Group Sessions

The results of group sessions can be exponentially more powerful than a single person working alone. Sometimes when I am demonstrating my work in front of a large audience, I may come across someone who does not seem to be responding to the energy.

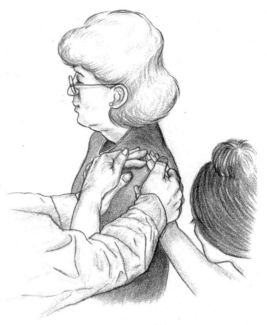

When this occurs, I'll send the non-responding person over to a couple of students who will usually be able to do what I could not.

When one person sandwiches their hands over an area that needs healing, they are establishing a powerful resonance between their hands and the area of pain. However, when two people are working on someone, instead of building a resonance between themselves and the person in pain, the practitioners are building a resonance with each other. That new and extraordinary resonance is often exponentially more powerful than working alone.

I really enjoy working in groups – perhaps it is because I am lazy, or perhaps because I like being effective. In any event, when you have a friend or client who does not seem to be responding, you might try doing a group session. Truly something magical happens when two or more are gathered.

There is a powerful way for two people to work together – we call it the Club Sandwich. The two practitioners will sandwich the area they want to work on with their hands. Each practitioner will have one hand on the client and one hand over the hand of the other practitioner.

I remember when my friend Paul called me and told me that his friend Rick had fallen off a seventeen-foot scaffolding. One of his ribs punctured a lung, and the doctors had to pump five pints of blood from his right lung to save his life. When Rick was released from the hospital about a week after the accident, he was barely able to walk, and was not able to turn or to bend his body. His breathing was incredibly painful and shallow in his right lung.

Since Paul had just finished my Quantum-Touch class about a week before the accident, I decided to do the session with his help. In order to increase the power of the session, we used a stacking-hands technique. I put one hand on Rick's chest, and I had Paul put one hand on Paul's back across from my hand. I put my other hand on top of Paul's hand, and he put his other hand on top of my hand. So each of us had one hand directly on Rick, and Paul had one hand on top of mine and I had one on top of his.

In this way Paul and I set up a new and very powerful resonance that Rick could use to heal himself. As the session progressed, Rick started moaning and bending from the torso. I joked with Rick that by the sound of things, either this felt very good or he was having great sex. He laughed, which caused him pain and said, "This is much better than sex." As we continued to work, his breathing became much more open and free. In about an hour he was able to bend and turn quite freely, when before he was tremendously stiff. The next day when Rick went back to his doctor, his doctor was amazed because Rick had 60 percent use of his right lung. The doctor inquired if Rick had done the coughing exercise that he had prescribed. Rick said that he had not, but that his friends had run energy into his lung. The doctor said something very interesting at that point. He said, "I don't want to hear about it." Rick then inquired if medicine was an empirical science, or a dogmatic religion. The doctor pondered this for a moment and repeated these thoughtful and memorable words, "I don't want to hear about it."

I encourage you to explore this area of the work. Whenever you can give a session with another trained Quantum-Touch practitioner, it is a great way to boost the effectiveness of your Quantum-Touch sessions, and it is a whole lot of fun.

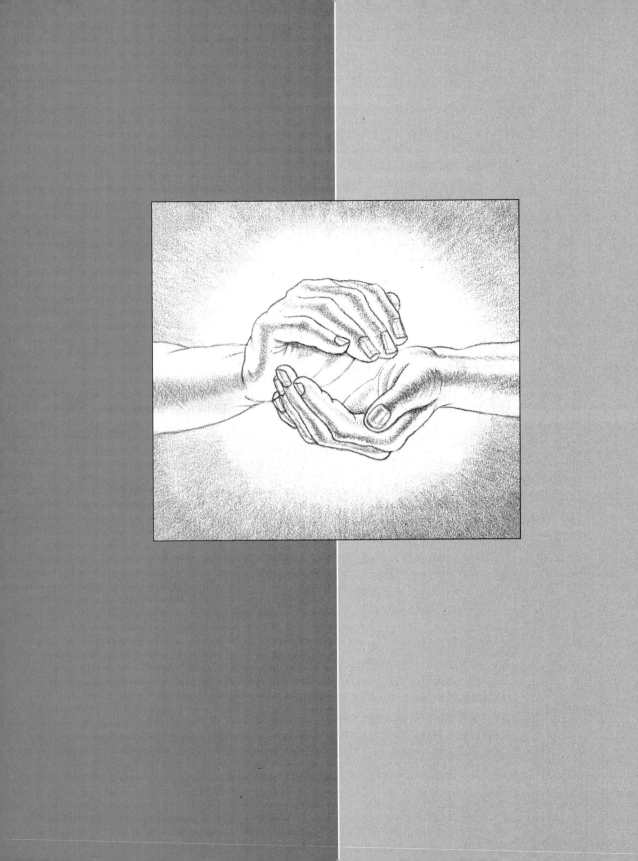

Chapter 6

Advanced Techniques

The depth, wonder, power, and brilliance of your love is not only more than you know, it is more than you could ever possibly imagine.

I recommend that you develop a strong foundation of skill and confidence with the beginning and intermediate techniques before working with the advanced ones. As you will see, it is not necessary that you use all the intermediate techniques; however, it is essential that you develop skill in using the beginning techniques as they become a strong foundation to the others. The intermediate and advanced techniques can further empower the strength of your healing work. The advanced techniques usually require skills that are naturally learned after you have obtained success using the beginning and intermediate ones. I strongly recommend that you use beginning and intermediate techniques for about twenty to fifty hours before trying the advanced ones. I should also let you know that there are many extraordinary healers simply using the beginning techniques by themselves and getting incredibly wonderful results. The most important thing is not how many of these techniques you know, but rather how much you practice and how skilled you become.

When I teach Quantum-Touch workshops, it is very exciting for me to get to this part of the class. By the time we start learning the advanced techniques, the level of enthusiasm in the room has become high, and we will have heard so many people tell of extraordinary healings that they have experienced or participated in.

The "advanced" exercises and techniques are built on a foundation of skills acquired from doing the basic and intermediate exercises and techniques. I urge you to develop a strong foundation of skills before you start working with these exercises. These techniques are generally more powerful than the basic and intermediate ones and require increased levels of skill or confidence that can be obtained through experience.

The "What You Love Most" Technique

(Also known as the "Julius Technique")

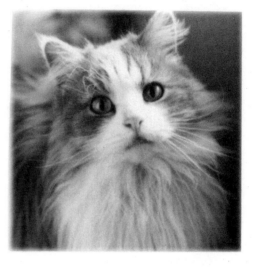

This is one of the easiest and most natural techniques. Over many years, I have repeatedly heard stories of people with no formal training in hands-on healing who suddenly felt inspired to do this work and astonished themselves by obtaining tremendously successful results. Later on, when they tried to do this again, they had no clue as to what had happened or how they had done it. In my opinion, the "what you love most" technique was probably the secret to their singular success.

When you can connect to the depths of your love, you have changed the vibration of your hands. My friend Billie has and adores about ten cats at any given time. All her cats are special and most wonderful and loving companions, but as she puts it, one of her cats makes her heart "bubble." This cat is named Julius, and he has the ability to give a look of exquisite adoration that is quite amazing (see photo). Billie has learned to access the love that she feels for this special cat to empower her healing sessions, and you can do the same. Gratitude, joy, and love are contagious.

I have placed this technique in the advanced section of the book, not because it is difficult, but because I wanted you to be completely sure that you knew that you did not have to use it in order to get wonderful results. When some of my students have tried to force themselves to use this technique, all they accomplished was making themselves quite uncomfortable in their efforts to do so. The secret to using the "what you love most" technique is to only use it when doing so requires no special effort to change your mood.

> *Your love can be harnessed to become*
> *a great and wonderful healing force.*

1. Let yourself remember and re-experience someone or something in your life that causes you to feel a tremendous sense of love, gratitude, happiness, or joy. Simply open your emotions to think of the person, situation, animal, plant, or whatever it is that lights and inspires your passion.

2. Let this emotion fill your body with as much tactile sensation as possible. Pay attention to where in your body you are feeling the emotion. For example, if you feel the love in your chest, feel it there with as much sensation as you can muster and let it spread through your body.

3. Run the tactile sensations of your love, joy, happiness, or gratitude out of your hands and combine it with the breathing techniques. It is as simple as that. Simply use your intention to move the tactile sensation of the emotion through your body and then out of your hands.

You can also use any other extremely positive emotion in place of love. Other emotions you can use to good advantage include enthusiasm, contentment, wonder, or inspiration.

Please do not try to force yourself to feel positive emotions, as this is not effective or even fun. Use your emotions that come easily, and only use this technique if you are in the mood to do so.

The Slope Breath

I discovered the slope breath because after twenty years I naturally found myself automatically doing it. It requires a level of skill that many beginners may find difficult.

Inhale with a one-four or two-six breath, and when you have finished inhaling, very slowly let the air out at the beginning of the exhalation. As you continue exhaling, gradually speed up the exhalation till you have exhaled the air to the count of four or six, depending on which breath you are doing. The exhalation gets faster and faster the more air you are exhaling, like the way your speed would accelerate if you were going down a slope. The trick to doing this technique well is to pay extremely close attention to the sensations in your hands. You will need to feel the sensations in your hands getting stronger and stronger as you exhale more and more air. An image to help you visualize what I'm describing is to imagine that you are blowing on a hot coal. The harder you exhale, the brighter the burning coal becomes.

I have placed this technique in the advanced section because it will be necessary to be able to clearly feel the intensity of sensation increasing in your hands as you exhale. Be sure to take full breaths and do not exhale longer than to the count of six.

Harmonic Toning

For those who love to use toning, harmonic toning is a great way to amplify the power of your Quantum-Touch sessions. As with other toning when using Quantum-Touch, be sure to complete your exhalations in no more than the count of six. With harmonic toning, you can mentally tone more than one note at a time to create harmonies. Experiment with various tones and vowel sounds to find the tones that have the greatest degree of sensation in your hands.

Another variation of this technique is to mentally tone a note and lift the pitch higher and higher until it is above hearing range. Don't be surprised if you can no longer imagine hearing it, since that is the idea. Then lift two other tones till they are also above hearing range and they are also in harmony with the first note. So now, you have three tones that are all in harmony with one another and all above hearing range. While you are doing this, imagine the health and well-being of the person you are working on. Imagine that there is a perfection that is expressing itself into their lives. Even though you may not know what that perfection is, it is expressing itself nevertheless. Then in this very pleasant (nonstressful) reverie, just lose yourself and keep the toning going. It is as if you were having a gentle dream.

The Funnel

This is a variation of spinning the energy. Imagine a cyclone of energy above your head. The point of the funnel goes into your head and all through your body, bringing you a tremendous source of energy. The important thing – the only thing that matters here – is that you can feel the funnel as a tactile sensation in your body. Just imagining a funnel is not enough here - it has to be something that you can actually feel in your body in order for this technique to be fully effective.

Feel the funnel of energy spinning through you while you are running energy. This technique can really amplify the energy of your healing sessions. **With all visualization techniques when using Quantum-Touch, the truly important thing is not what you see, but rather that you can have strong tactile sensations in your body and hands as a result of the visualization. Remember, it is all about sensation.**

The Amplified Resonance Technique

See chapter 12, page 179.

Working with Chakras
Eight through Twelve

Many people have heard of and worked with the seven major chakras of the body. Less well known are chakras eight through twelve, which I learned from Lazaris. If you have enjoyed the chakra technique in chapter five, I think you will really love working with these other chakras. Now that you have become skilled at getting chakras one through seven spinning, you can raise the energy of your Quantum-Touch sessions further by learning to work with chakras eight through twelve. Use the same meditative technique to spin each chakra one by one and to run this energy out of your hands. Many people have told me that using chakras eight through twelve has opened them up to a greater sense of spiritual connection during their sessions, and sometimes incredible successes. *Remember to use one of the breathing techniques during this exercise.*

Eighth Chakra

Symbolically, the eighth chakra represents probable realities and the astral plane and can be contacted below the feet. Imagine a ball of blazing and brilliant white light about eight or ten inches below your feet. Get the ball spinning in whichever direction feels good to you. The important thing is not only that you imagine that it is spinning, but that you can actually feel some physical sensation from it spinning.

Ninth Chakra

Symbolically the ninth chakra represents possible realities as well as the home of your higher self and is located above the crown of your head. Imagine a ball of blazing and brilliant white light about eight or ten inches above your head. Get the ball spinning in whichever direction feels good to you. Don't just imagine that it is spinning, but feel physical sensation from it spinning.

Tenth, Eleventh, and Twelfth Chakras

Symbolically, the tenth chakra represents what is truly real, beyond the illusion that we experience. The eleventh chakra represents the soul and spirit. The twelfth chakra represents your personal relationship to God, Universe, Goddess, All That Is, Great Spirit, or whatever you choose to use.

The tenth chakra is located about eight inches above the ninth chakra. Repeat the directions as in the ninth chakra description. The eleventh is about eight or ten inches above the tenth. The twelfth is placed another eight or ten inches above the eleventh. Follow the same procedure to get them spinning while using your breathing techniques.

Once you have experienced chakras eight through twelve spinning, there are two popular approaches to working with the chakras. The first approach is to work your way up chakras one through twelve and run the energy out of your hands with each chakra. Spend a longer time when you find one that causes you to feel more sensations in your hands. This is an indication that there is a greater resonance there. The second approach is a bit more challenging. This is to get all twelve chakras spinning at once and then run the energy out of your hands. As long as you bring strong tactile sensations to your hands as a result of spinning the chakras, either technique will work quite well. Some people have found that by simply getting the twelfth chakra spinning well, it can cause all the others to start spinning as well.

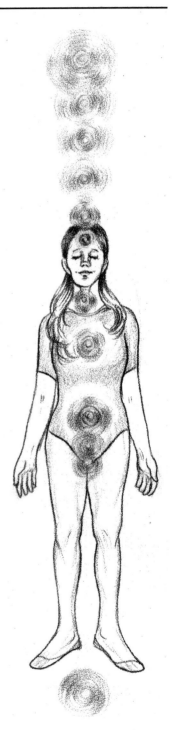

Unless you know better, I suggest you run energy from all the chakras. You can spin them one at a time or all at once and then run the energy out your hands.

Asking for Help

For those of you who like to work with your higher self, angels, guides, or spiritual teachers, it can only improve things to ask for help during your sessions. Tapping into feelings of your own spirituality can only raise your own vibration, and the positive expectation and help that is received can only make things better as well. To make this work even more effectively, let yourself feel the hand of whomever you called for help. Let yourself feel the tactile sensations of his or her hands over yours and then feel the gratitude for the help.

Raising Expectation

In 1980, I used to spend hours sitting with Bob Rasmusson to try to understand why he was able to run the energy so much more powerfully than anyone else. I would ask him every question that I could think of to uncover his secrets. I believe that one of those secrets had to do with expectation.

I have purposely chosen to place this technique in this chapter because I have seen people misuse it to their own detriment. Holding a high level of expectation about the outcome of a session does clearly raise your resonance and can be a powerful factor in shaping the outcome of a session. Yet asking people to hold a high level of expectation before they are ready to do so may only put them into a place of self-doubt. Self-doubt, by the way, is not one of the preferred states to be in when doing this work.

Even if you have not reached a place where you know how wonderful Quantum-Touch is yet, you can hold the belief that anything is possible. Since beliefs precede expectations, you can choose to hold the belief that healing could be possible, that the body knows how to heal itself, that there is a perfection that the body can approach. If all else fails, you can approach a session with a completely neutral expectation of "I don't know what will happen." Even a neutral expectation can work wonderfully well. The main point here is to raise your level of expectation as high as you can honestly raise it without slipping into self-doubt.

Healing the Past

The first time I used this technique, I was simply amazed and overjoyed by the results. It had come to my attention that most children in Western civilization are not held as much as children who come from many undeveloped or primitive cultures. Jean Liedloff, an anthropologist who wrote a great book called *The Continuum Concept,* wrote that in some primitive societies the children never ever hit one another. In these societies, the babies were carried everywhere and not put down. She speculated that the children had an excess of energy that they had to release and that when the children were held, they gave some of that energy to their parents. When children were not held, they become aggressive and violent. I suspect that a great deal of the dissatisfaction and alienation so painfully visible in Western civilization may have roots in the severe touch deprivation of its people. We have become wealthy enough to become alienated and isolated.

One day I decided to meditate on healing my past when I was an infant and to give myself some of the physical touch I did not receive. During this meditation, I had mentally gone back in time and imagined that I was holding myself as an infant. Since I was holding this little baby in my hands, I decided to start running energy into the baby. In a few seconds after I started running energy, I had an experience that I have never had before or since. Suddenly, a huge surge of energy shot through me. My spine spontaneously shifted like a whip, causing me to suddenly sit up a bit straighter. I don't know what happened, but it was quite unexpected and dramatic.

The technique is very easy. Simply get very relaxed into a meditative state and imagine that you are going back in time. Hold the young version of yourself at any age you like. While you are holding the baby or child, just start to run energy out of your hands and do the breathing as with any other healing session.

Combine Multiple Techniques

With practice you will be able to combine techniques together to great advantage. The combining of techniques requires more focus on the part of the practitioner, and ultimately, the more you can give yourself to the process, the more effective it becomes. Combining your favorite techniques can allow you to creatively add to the work and to find out what suits you best.

Here are a few examples of how you can combine techniques while running the energy out your hands and continuing the breath work:

- Tone while spinning the energy as in the vortex technique or the funnel technique. The higher the tone, the faster the energy spins.

- Spin the chakras one at a time while using the "what you love most" technique.

- Enter the tissue being healed as described in chapter 12, while toning and holding a high expectation.

I think you get the idea of what I'm talking about. Go ahead and make up combinations that you like. Have fun!

Keys to Always Remember

Trusting the process is essential. Healing work may cause temporary pain or other distressing symptoms that are all part of the healing. The life-force and healing process work with complexity and wisdom that are beyond our conception or comprehension. If problems arise, keep running the energy.

- Keep your breathing going.

- Connect your breathing to the sensations in your hands.

- No one can really heal anyone else. The person in need of healing is the healer. The practitioner simply holds a resonance to allow that to happen.

- The energy follows the natural intelligence of the body to do the necessary healing. The practitioner pays attention to "body intelligence" and "chases the pain."

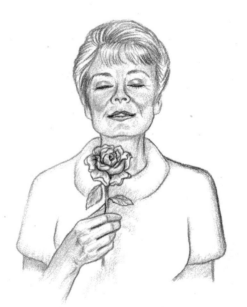

More Q & A

Do I have to keep counting to keep track of each of my breaths?

No, the count is just a guideline to keep you breathing, and are about one second in length. Once you have a sense of doing the breathing, you can just settle into a rhythm. It is very important to maintain awareness of what you are feeling in your hands. With each breath you can track how the sensations in your hands change. This can be very useful information, and in and of itself, it can become a useful reminder to keep you breathing. In time, each person finds their own rythym of breathing that works best.

Have you ever been scared by what happens during a session?

There have been a few occasions when people have had a strong reaction to the energy. In retrospect, it was because their body was going through an extremely rapid healing process.

On one occasion, I was demonstrating the usefulness of Quantum-Touch for treating repetitive strain injuries such as carpal tunnel syndrome. I was at a large Silicon Valley company that had a few thousand employees. The woman who had invited me (call her Jane) was the health director of the company, and she had the director of security in the room to witness the work I was doing.

Jane seemed to be acting like a nervous New Yorker who had just had six cups of coffee. Before I started the sessions on the four people with painful wrist conditions, I (foolishly) decided it would be helpful if I gave Jane an experience of the work. I noticed that the back of her occipital ridge was extraordinarily uneven. One of the people with wrist problems was an engineer, and pressing her thumbs against Jane's occipital ridge, she confirmed that the ridge was quite far from being even.

Standing behind Jane I touched my thumbs to her occipital ridge, and my fingers went along the sides of her head. A few seconds later, I noticed that she was leaning forward – next thing I knew, Jane's knees were buckling. I quickly reached under her arms to catch her and help her to the floor.

So there was Jane, lying on the floor with her eyes wide open. The security director picked up her walkie-talkie and yelled, Code Blue – emergency in conference room #4. The paramedics should be along shortly," she announced. During this time I continued to run energy into Jane's head. In about a minute, Jane woke up and told us she felt great, and very refreshed, but she wondered what she was doing on the floor. The engineer checked the position of her occipital ridge and was shocked to see that the bones appeared to be totally aligned.

The point of the story is that when the energy works in an unpredictable and even disturbing manner, I have found that more and not less energy is the answer.

To follow up on the story, Jane went to a doctor the next day to get checked out. The doctor asked her, "How hard did he press into the back of your head?" She explained that I had barely touched the back of her head. The doctor then proclaimed, "He couldn't have possibly done anything to you then."

I had been hoping to be strong enough to "knock them off their feet." I just never actually thought that I would really knock her off her feet. Now when I demonstrate moving occipital bones, I like people seated.

How do you decide which of the various techniques to use at any particular time?

I have provided you with more techniques than you need. Simply find the ones that you enjoy using the most and go with those. I never intended that people should use all the various approaches. The important thing is to find out what works for you and then have fun. Once you understand the basic principles of the work, you can start to find original ways of running the energy. As long as you are doing the breathing and connecting it to the energy, everything you try will work. Some approaches will clearly work better for you than others. This is a system that is meant to grow and evolve. Write to us and tell us what you have learned and we may include it on our web site at *www.quantumtouch.com*.

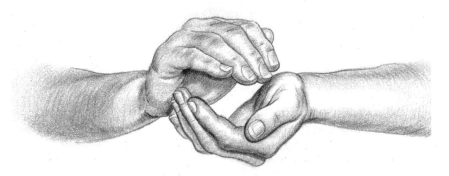

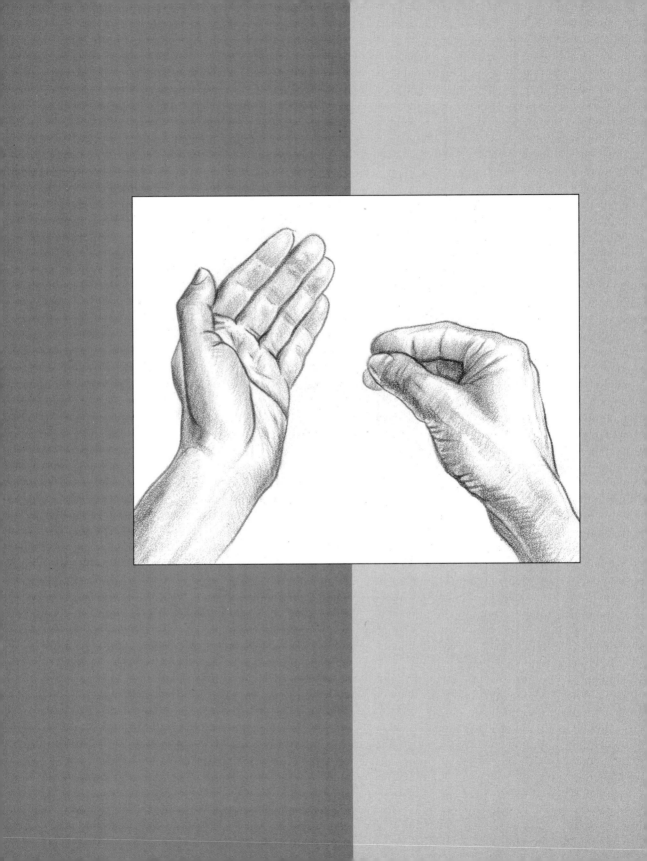

Chapter 7

Altering Posture
with Energy

On the Brink

*We now stand on the brink of extraordinary
breakthroughs in the art of hands-on healing.
Human abilities that heretofore may well have
been considered "science fiction" are in fact
quite real and can withstand the
rigors of scientific scrutiny.*

Confronting the Impossible

A few years back, I gave a lecture at a large conference in San Francisco. I had explained to the audience how easy it is to learn to use Quantum-Touch, and that among numerous sorts of healing events, bones will spontaneously move back into alignment with only a light touch – even cranial bones.

After my lecture was over, a man approached me and stated, "I've got a Ph.D. in physiology, and I know that you can't possibly move the cranial bones because they are rigidly fused in place!" I responded by saying, "I'm so glad to meet you. Come here; let me show you what I'm talking about." Within moments, I found someone who had been in my audience whose cranial bones were severely uneven.

I placed my thumbs on both sides of her occipital ridge, pressed up on the back of her head, and saw that one side was much higher than the other. "What do you see here?" I asked him. He placed his thumbs in the same position and pressed up. After a bit of analysis he said, "The left side looks higher." "How much higher?" I asked. He placed his thumbs back on her occipital ridge, measured again even more carefully and said, "At least one half an inch, maybe five-eighths of an inch." I told him that that was exactly what I saw. I then lightly touched my thumbs to the base of her occipital ridge, placed my fingertips on the sides of her head and started to run the energy. After about fifteen seconds, I asked him to check again. He rolled his eyes incredulously and measured her. This time, he kept measuring and measuring for about a full minute. He finally announced that the occipital ridge looked completely even. "Do you have any interest in researching this?" I asked. And with that, he said, "No, I work on amphibians." And then he just walked away.

I'll now show you that you can easily do what conventional science claims to be quite impossible. My warning to you is that when you discover that you can do this, you may have to stretch your beliefs a bit. This can be uncomfortable for some people. I'm not asking you to change your beliefs, but merely to follow the directions and honestly see what happens.

If you have practiced the exercises in chapter 3, you are ready to proceed. At this point, you should be able to:

- Feel the energy flow through your body and into your hands.

- Do the breathing techniques.

- Connect your breathing to your sensations.

Keep in Mind

When you run the energy with the intent of altering someone's posture, there are some important things to keep in mind:

This sort of manipulation of the skeletal structure is so harmonious, the bones seem to "melt" back into alignment. You rarely hear any clicking or crunching as with many chiropractic maneuvers.

- You don't need to decide where or if the bones should move – the body figures that out. The person's body intelligence decides what should happen. More often than not, the person's body will "choose" to put the bones back into place. For reasons about which I can only speculate, the body really seems to like having its structure aligned.

- Bones will move more easily if you use a light touch. Do not try to direct or push or use force, as this is counterproductive. People have become so conditioned to try to dominate situations by use of force. This is one case where force is not only not called for, but ineffective. Be sure your hands are very relaxed. Many of my students, especially people who have done various kinds of massage or deep tissue work, have a strong tendency to rigidly hold tension in their hands. Let your hands get soft and relaxed. Energy flows more easily through them when you are not tense.

- Structural corrections happen more easily when a person is sitting or standing. For some reason, structural realignment happens most fluidly when people are upright. This is not to say you can never effect change when a person is lying down, but it is easier when a person is seated or standing. This is very convenient since just about anywhere you go, you can find a place to stand and, in most cases, to sit as well.

- When you run energy, many sorts of healing can take place, and only part of that process causes the bones to move. Since altering posture with a light touch is so dramatic and unexpected, I like to demonstrate it to groups. Many who observe this will naturally assume that structural realignment is what this work is all about. The movement of the bones is like the tip of an iceberg because there is so much more going on below the surface. Since we are not easily aware of the myriad changes taking place on a cellular level, we say that the bones move because it is something we can clearly see.

- Sometimes the bones move quickly, sometimes slowly, and occasionally not at all. There are times when the body is very happy to have the structure the way it is, and no matter how much energy you put into the system, it will remain structurally the same. It is only common sense that you can't fix what ain't broke. When treating people with chronic back problems, you may be able to observe structural changes happening within a few minutes, or it could take ten, twenty, or even thirty minutes before the changes become visible. In most cases, some postural adjustments will happen within two to five minutes, and sometimes within seconds.

If you have successfully done the exercises in chapter 3, then, despite the fact that you may adamantly not believe it, you are indeed ready!

There are two places in the body where the bones move most visibly and easily: the hips and the occipital ridge. For the purpose of being able to see that you can alter posture with a light touch, let's start with the hips.

Measuring and Altering Hip Position

Find someone who has one hip higher than the other. Some people really do have a long leg, and this technique will not correct that. The vast majority of people can be adjusted if they are out of alignment.

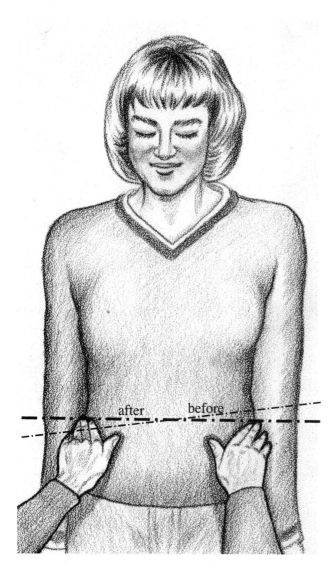

1. Place your fingertips on the crest of their ileum (the top of the hip bone) and press down lightly and evenly on both sides. In order to see if one side is higher than the other, you must have your eyes level with the place you are measuring. I constantly have to remind students to get down on one knee so they can check to see if the hips are level. In many cases, the difference will be quite obvious, and in other cases the difference is insignificant. I suggest that for the purpose of testing this for yourself, you find some people who are clearly high on one side.

2. Once you have determined which side is higher and how much higher it is, take the palms of your hands, and place them gently on the crest of the ileum. Do not press down, but simply start

running the energy. Do a full body sweep, feel full sensations gathering in your hands and do one of the breathing techniques. I would suggest for this demonstration that a 1-4 breath should work quite well. Keep the breathing going and run the energy into the ileum for one to ten minutes. Sometimes the bones move almost immediately from the second they are touched; other times it takes longer.

3. Be sure to ask the person you are working on if they can feel anything or have any interesting sensations. Many people can feel the energy almost the second you start to run it.

4. Follow the same directions on the back side of the ileum that you used on the front. The ileum is a surprisingly complex structure, in that it can turn sideways, up and down, and all sorts of

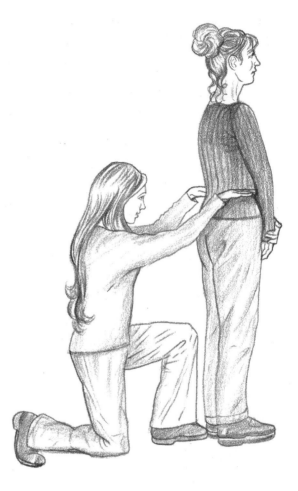

Be sure that your eyes are level with your hands as you measure the position of the hips.

combined ways. Sometimes one side will be high in the front and the other side will be high in the back. It is always a good idea to balance both the front and back sides of the ileum.

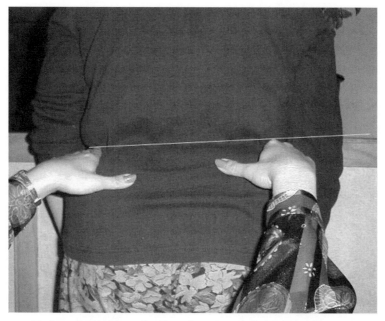

Before and after adjusting the hips, it is common to see adjustments such as this, or even more dramatic results.

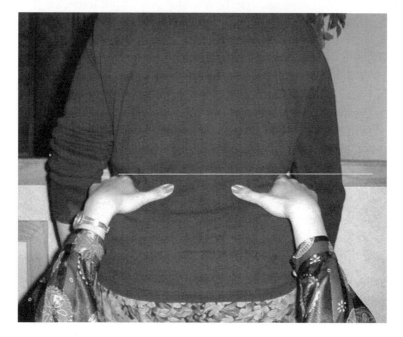

Adjusting the Hips Front to Back

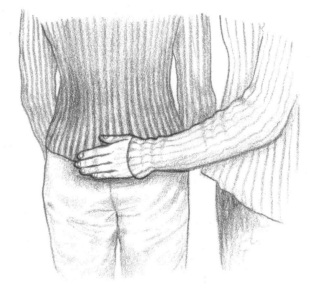

The hips can also be adjusted from front to back,
as illustrated by these two pictures.

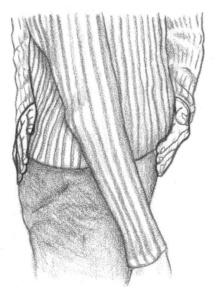

Transforming Structural Alignment

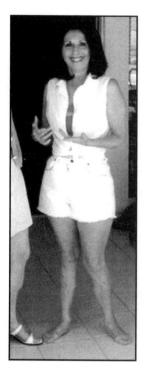

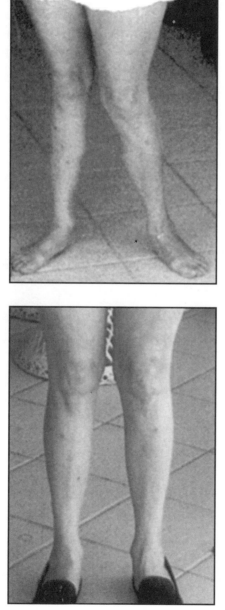

Roberta's leg had been misaligned for six years due to Multiple Sclerosis (left).

The lower pictures show the dramatic improvement due to a single Quantum-Touch session. (below) She reports that her legs feel fine, the change is lasting, and she is walking much better now.

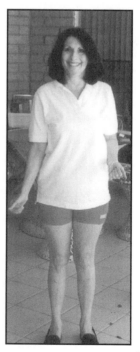

The more we use Quantum-Touch, we become increasingly aware that we don't know the limits of this work.

Measuring and Altering the Position of the Occipital Ridge

Based on more than twenty years of experience with this phenomenon, the human body has a tremendous desire to realign the skeletal structure and especially the cranium. The occipital ridge is probably the easiest structure in the body to move with life-force energy. Ironically, it is considered the structure least likely to move by physiologists and the medical profession. For whatever reasons, the body's innate intelligence really wants you to have your head on straight.

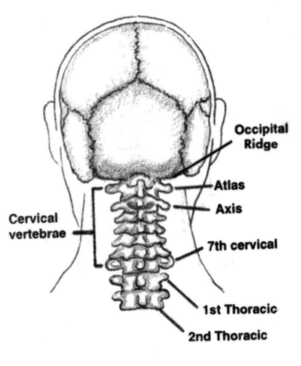

The first time I had this done, I had an experience I will never forget. This was the first session that I was to receive from my teacher, Bob Rasmusson. I remember sitting on the end of the table and looking out an open window. Bob placed his thumbs lightly on the base of my occipital ridge and suddenly, the whole window appeared to tip sideways about 35 degrees. A moment later, it straightened out. I think that when the occipital ridge moved, the orbitals, which hold the eyes in place, moved as well, causing my brain to temporarily see the window at a severe angle. In about one half of a second, my brain was able to recalibrate and make things appear level again.

Over the last twenty years, I have observed this shift of cranial bones happen about fifty times. If I find someone who has their occipital ridge far out of alignment, I will ask them to keep their eyes open for the next

Temporal Suture

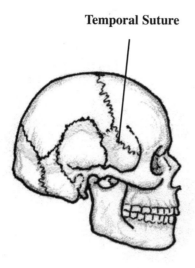

thirty seconds to see if they have this experience. About one out of ten people who are very far out of alignment will see it happen. So as to not project my expectation, I have been careful not to explain why I want them to keep their eyes open until the bones have moved back into place, as I wanted them to have their own experience.

I have been told by chiropractors that altering the cranial bones is an excellent way to get the body to start to realign the entire spine. Undoubtedly, there are other benefits to doing this move, since the body seems so determined that it should happen. Some people have told me that it relieved or eliminated chronic headaches or sinus pain. Generally, more healing work is appropriate for these conditions.

1. If you slide your thumbs up both sides of the neck and press in lightly, you will eventually come to the base of the cranium. The tissue there is not as soft as the neck because you are now pressing up against bone.

2. Try to place your thumbs so they are equidistant from the center of the head, with one thumb on each side. There is usually a little ridge on both sides where your thumbs conveniently fit.

3. Do not let the person you are measuring move their hair out of the way. The act of lifting hair will angle their head and interfere with your ability to measure whether the occipital ridge is even or not. Instead, place your thumbs over the hair and press up on the hair.

4. Look closely at the positions of your thumbs to determine if they are even with one another. Adjust your body so your eyes are level with the occipital ridge. You must have your eyes level with

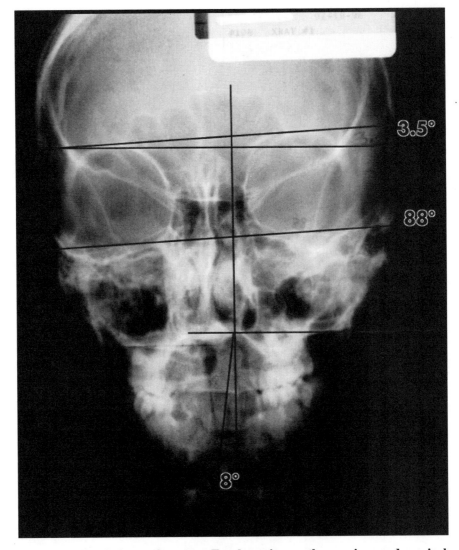

An x-ray taken before a Quantum-Touch session on the cranium and cervical vertebrae; note how the axis vertebrae points 8⁰ to the left nostril.

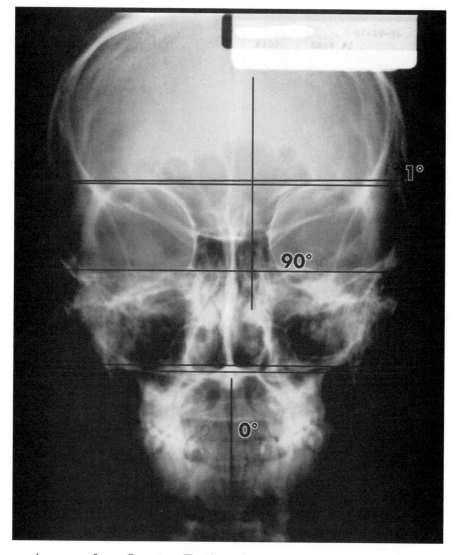

An x-ray after a Quantum-Touch session on the cranium and cervical vertebrae; note how the axis vertebrae now points up vertically.

your thumbs if you hope to get a good reading. Admittedly, some of my students seem to be able to do this naturally, and others never become competent.

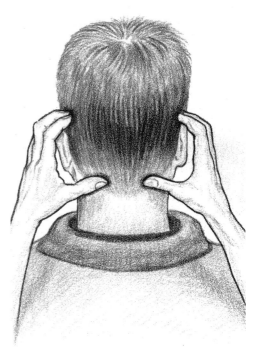

5. Have the client seated when you do this. The power of this move can be quite remarkable. I have seen one woman pass out for a couple minutes and a few other people nearly faint. Those rare individuals are more likely to faint if they are standing when you do this. These extreme reactions are the body's way of finding a new place of balance. The people with these reactions always felt much better after they had the session.

6. While a client is in a seated position, lightly touch your thumbs to the base of the occipital ridge and rest your fingertips on the sides of his or her head. Run the energy out of your fingertips and use one of the breathing techniques. The cranial bones will usually move in the first five to twenty seconds that you do this. There is also benefit to doing this move longer.

If you have been able to do the energy exercises in chapter 3 and have worked with a few people, by now you should have seen that bones do in fact move. I suggest that you savor this experience.

Starting a Session

When beginning a session, it is often a great idea to use the following Quantum-Touch techniques. If you spend a minute or two on each of these positions, it will help to free up your client's energy and accelerate their healing process.

Balance the occipital ridge (p.130)

Adjust the neck (p.139)

Adjust the hips from the front (p.121)

Adjust the hips from the back (p.123)

Adjust from the psoas to sciatica point (p.142-143)

Incidentally, the chiropractors are right, in that the body wants the bones into their proper alignment. You can see for yourself that this is not a theory, because when you run energy, the bones will spontaneously adjust themselves. (p118)

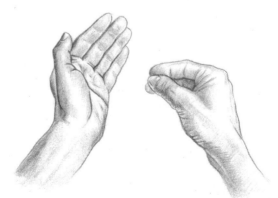

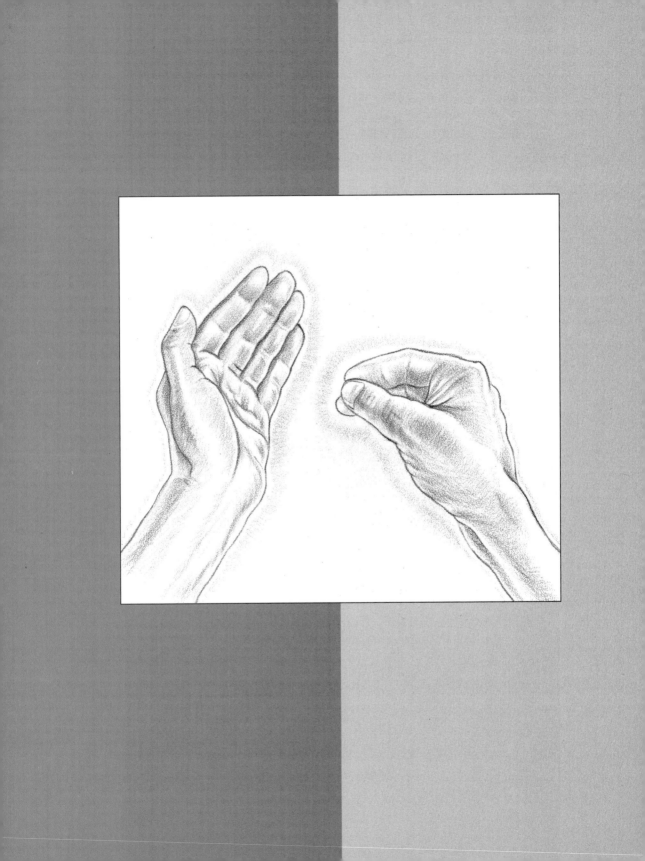

Chapter 8

Working on Back and Neck Problems

Love can unite your breath with intent, like focusing a light and causing fire to ignite.

The most common problems I see in clients are neck and back pain. Since these conditions are so prevalent, I decided to write a separate chapter about them. Be aware that working on this sort of pain is only one of the many highly effective applications of Quantum-Touch. Over the years, I have found it highly gratifying to observe new students being able to assist in alleviating neck pain, lower back pain, and sciatica in their very first sessions.

If you have practiced the exercises in chapter 3, can feel the energy during full body sweeps, and can link that energy with your breath to the sensations in your hands, you are ready to learn to do remarkable work on a wide variety of spinal problems.

Work on Both Sides of the Vertebrae

The first thing to do when you are dealing with someone with neck or back pain is to work on both sides of the spine. The ideal place to place your hands or fingertips is at the outer ends of each vertebra. It is ineffective to try to work from the front of the body as you will be adjusting the energy in all the organs as well as the spine. The general rule is that the closer you can place your hands to the exact spot were the pain resides, the more effective you will be. Using a tripod hand position on both sides of the spine creates a powerful resonance to allow vertebrae to spontaneously slide back into correct alignment.

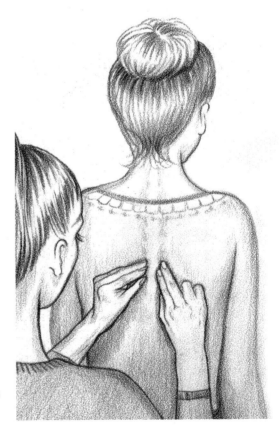

Compensation

When you observe someone's spine from the side, you see that the spine is not straight, but gently curves in and out as you go from the top of the neck to the tip of the tailbone. These curves are quite well placed to provide support and balance for the spine.

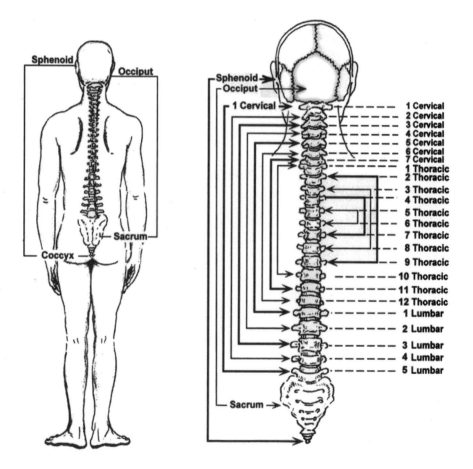

When there is pain or injury to one part of the spine, the body often compensates by placing stress on other parts as well. This makes sense if you think of the spine as a complete structure, rather than as a series of sections. There is a reflexive sort of reaction between the top of the spine and the lower part of the spine. In most cases when there is injury or pain, the spine will compensate as a whole unit.

If you encounter a person who has pain in a lower part of the back, it is usually necessary to work on the neck also. And similarly, if someone has pain in his or her neck, it is usually necessary to work on the lower back also. Before the spine is going to readjust itself, it needs to "know" that it is safe to change its position. Before the neck will safely move itself into alignment, it may need to know that the lower back is also able to move as well. In this manner, the whole spine can find a new balance in which to function.

General Points to Keep in Mind for Neck and Back Pain

- Ask the person in pain to point to exactly where he or she is hurting, place your hands there and run the energy. Don't make assumptions about where the pain is. The closer you can be to the exact point, the faster the effect will be.

- Use a tripod hand position or the palms of your hands when touching your client. The tripod is great if you are comfortable; otherwise use the palms, thumbs, or fingertips. Remember, you can run the energy out of any part of your body if you apply your intention.

- Place your hands in the most comfortable position you can find. I suggest you move around if you are not comfortable and look for a position where you are comfortable.

- Do not use any force or pressure in your touch. Keep your hands relaxed and let the energy do the work.

- Work on people's necks and backs when they are seated or standing. Standing generally works best on the lower back, and seated works well for the neck. If there has been injury to the tissue, it is probably best that the person be seated or lying down. Above all, be sure that the person you are working on is comfortable.

- Keep your breathing going and use any of the energy techniques you choose. Be sure to connect your breathing to the sensation of energy.

- Hold the points as long as necessary. Pay attention to the sensations in your hands as described in chapter 3. It may take as little as a few minutes or it may take repeated one-hour sessions to assist your client. The easiest way to know is to give the energy and to ask the person how he or she is doing.

- Chase the pain or sensation. Keep a dialogue going with the person you are working with and have them tell you if the pain has shifted or moved. Change the position of your hands to follow the pain or sensation.

- Sometimes putting energy into the body can cause pain temporarily. This has shown repeatedly itself to be a very good sign that healing is happening. This pain is usually very short-lived. Should pain arise, encourage your client to breathe deeply into the pain while it is still there.

- Amplify the power of your work by having the person you are working on breathe deeply too.

- For longer sessions, when there are areas of particular difficulty, you can have a person on a massage table face up or down, and place your hands over the spine. You can also have the person on the massage table face up, and place your hands under the spine.

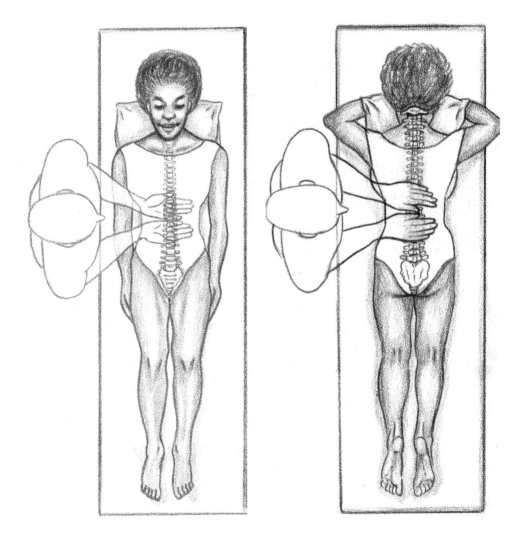

Working with Neck Pain

- Run energy into the occipital ridge for a minute or two with the fingertips on the sides of the head along the line of the temporal suture. (see p. 127)

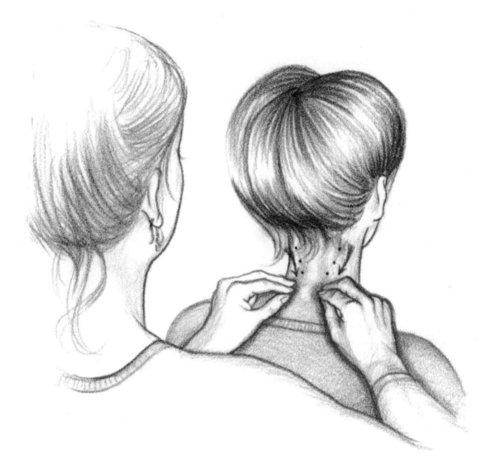

- Be sure to work on both sides of the vertebrae in the neck, paying particular attention to any areas that are in pain.

- You may need to pay particular attention to the atlas, axis, and seventh cervical vertebrae. (see p. 119)

- Be sure to run energy on areas of tightness or pain in the client's lower back, which may correspond to the neck pain.

- Adjust their hips, front and back, as shown in the previous chapter.

- Keep a dialogue going and chase the pain or sensation.

Working with Lower Back Pain

- Adjust the hips on both the front and the back as described previously.

- Run energy into the areas of pain.

- Run energy into the neck, especially areas of tightness or of pain. Follow the guidelines for working on the neck as listed in the previous section.

- Keep a dialogue going and chase the pain or sensation.

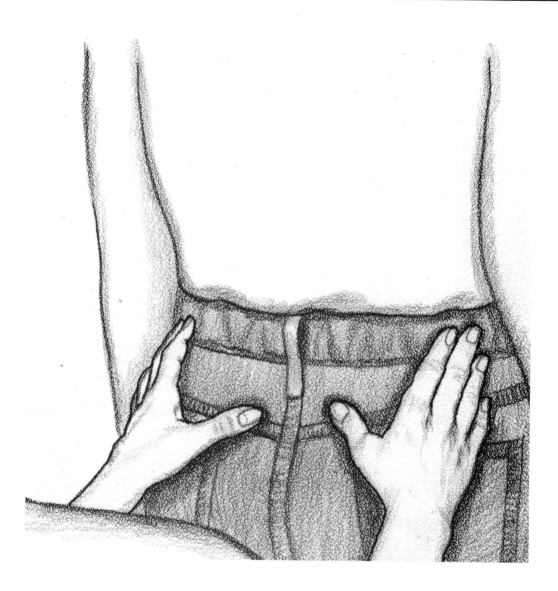

Working with Sciatica

Follow the guidelines for working with the lower back with these additions:

- Use your thumbs and give special attention to the areas of the buttocks that are illustrated here. Work on both sides of the buttocks and give more attention to the side that is in pain.

- Run energy into any area down the leg or in the foot that is experiencing pain. Go ahead and chase the pain or sensation anywhere that it takes you.

- Work on any other area that is experiencing pain during or after the session.

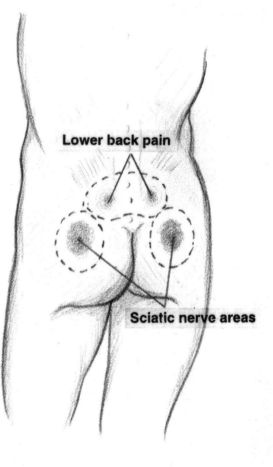

Lower back pain

Sciatic nerve areas

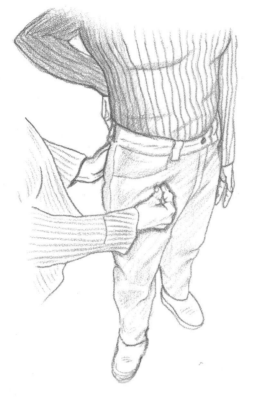

Psoas Sciatica Release

This is a great way to release the psoas muscle and help sciatica pain. Place one hand over the psoas, as shown, and the other hand over the sciatica point, as illustrated on the previous page.

Mid-back Pain

When there are problems in the middle of the back, you will often need to do some release work on the neck and the lower back. You can run as follows:

- Run energy into the occipital ridge and the neck.

- Run energy into the lower back and balance the hips.

- Work on the area that is in pain.

These simple guidelines will work wonders on most back pain caused by misalignment and injury. Of course, this is not the intended treatment for back pain due to kidney problems.

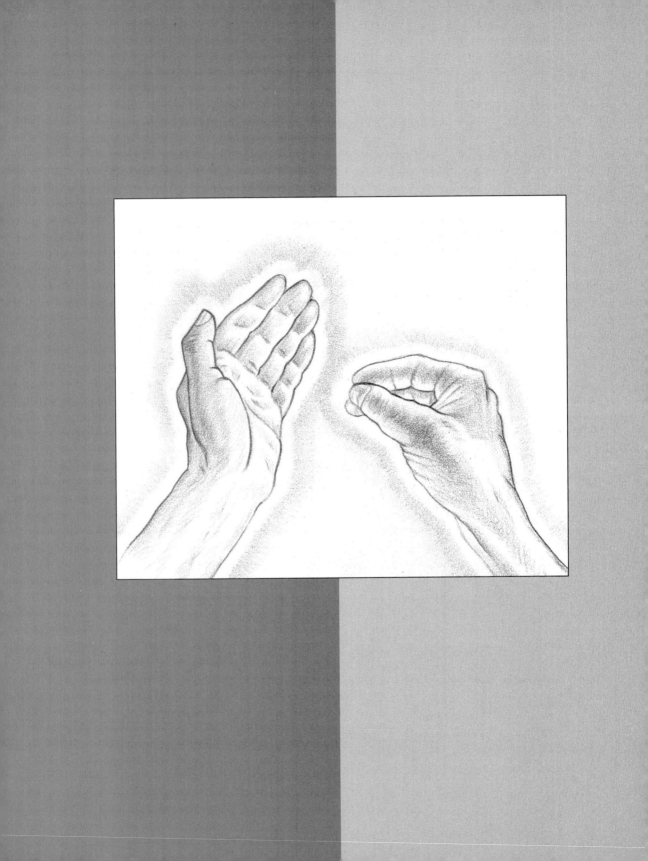

Chapter 9

Working Throughout the Body

*Open your eyes, pause to wonder, and
stand rapt in awe as you behold the
true nature of your gifts.*

Healing Hands

Have you ever wondered why people will immediately and automatically breathe deeply and put their hands on whatever part of their body was just injured? It seems that this action is universal and built into our neural hardware. Perhaps some part of us instinctively knows that this is a way for us to assist ourselves and others when in pain. It's funny, but after doing this work for over two decades, whenever I'm around someone who is in a lot of pain, I now have an immediate and automatic response – I start running the energy. I feel it surging throughout my body and into my hands. This may be a function of compassion or just conditioning, but perhaps this is a natural human response to seeing another in need.

Before we jump off into a wide variety of ways to place your hands, I thought it would be a good idea to give you a little perspective on working with hand positions. Over the years, I have observed some students manage to become upset and even overwhelmed by the thought of having to know exactly where to place their hands to be effective. This is understandable, since most subjects that are taught have become overly difficult and complicated with a specialized language so that only highly paid professionals will know what is being discussed. With hands-on healing in general, and particularly with Quantum-Touch, this is not so.

If you are ever in doubt as to where to place your hands, the easiest thing to do, and one which covers a multitude of problems, is simply to do what I showed you in chapter 3: sandwich the area that is in pain or needs to be healed between your two hands. The vast majority of conditions can be handled by sandwiching.

The Basic Hand Sandwich (Hold the mayo)

Sandwiching means that you have one hand on one side and the other hand on the other side of the part of the body you are treating.

The most important thing to remember is this: If the position that you have placed your hands is not optimal, in the vast majority of occasions, the person you are working on will feel sensations or pain move to another part of their body. If you keep an open dialogue with the person you are working on, they can tell you about other places to put your hands. This is one example of where trusting the process can be highly useful.

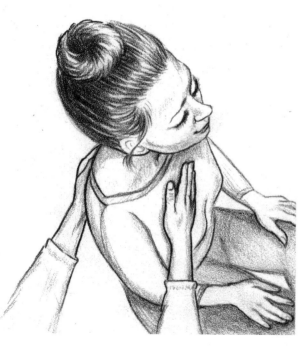

You truly could place one hand on the top of the head and the other hand on their knee and eventually get good results since the body will direct the life-force energy to where it should go. You will, however, get better results if you can place your hands as close as possible to the exact point that is experiencing pain or difficulty. So here are the basic things to remember about sandwiching, and then I'll show you some hand positions that are somewhat less obvious.

- Surround the part of the body that needs healing with your hands as close as possible to and on both sides of the problem you are working on. Go directly to the specific area if you can. Use common sense, of course. That is, don't put your hands into a wound or touch a burn. Surrounding the problem can mean placing your hands above and below or on either side of the point where you choose to focus the energy.

- Use your fingertips or tripod for putting energy around very small areas. Concentrating the energy works very well in such cases. This also helps you get your hands closer to the center of the area that needs healing.

- Chase the pain. Maintain a dialogue with the person you are working on and follow their sensations or pain around the body.

- Make sure that your body is comfortable while you are working.

- Keep the breathing going throughout the session.

Running Energy Directly On or Near the Surface

There are occasions when sandwiching is not as effective as running energy directly over the affected tissue of the body. Examples of places you would be more effective working directly over the tissue include topical problems like bee stings, poison oak, and burns. You can also treat eyes, sinuses, gums, kidneys, and adrenals. The principle is that you want to work on tissue that is not too far below the skin.

The field from your hands placed directly over the body will do wonderful work when it does not have to travel more than a few inches. If the energy does have to go more than a few inches, then sandwiching is the preferred position for your hands.

Since I am not there with you as you practice, I'll have to settle for nagging at you from a distance. **Keep Breathing!**

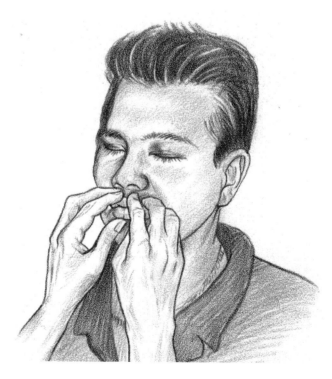

Specific Conditions

Headaches

Headaches are probably one of the more common problems you will encounter, and in most cases, even migraines can be dealt with effectively. I recommend that the person you are working with be either seated or lying down. Of course, be sure that your body is comfortable in each position you are working.

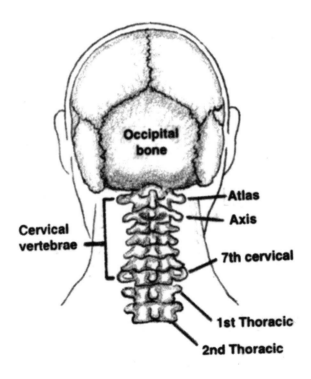

- Sandwich the head surrounding the area of pain.

- Balance the occipital ridge. (see p. 126)

- Run energy into the sutures. (see p. 185)

- You may also need to run energy into the atlas and axis.

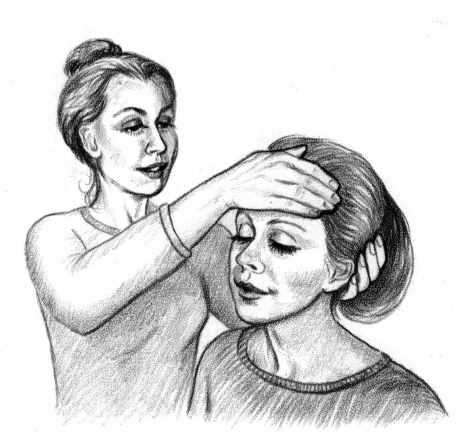

Eye Problems

Simply put your palms over the eyes and run the energy right in. Be sure not to press down on the eyes – let the energy do the work. Be patient, as it may take repeated sessions to make good progress. I've seen many cases where a person's vision has improved, at least temporarily.

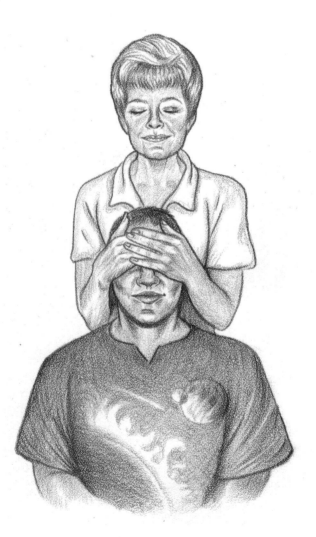

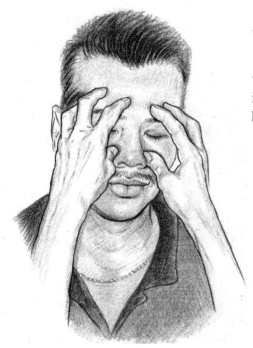

Sinus Problems

Sinus problems have often responded very quickly to running energy directly into them. Use fingertips or palms of hands.

Temporal-Mandibular Joint (TMJ)

Use a tripod hand position and place your fingertips right on the joint. You can tell if you are in the right place because the TMJ is a bony surface that moves when the mouth is opened or closed. In most cases the energy can relieve pain or tightness in the joint.

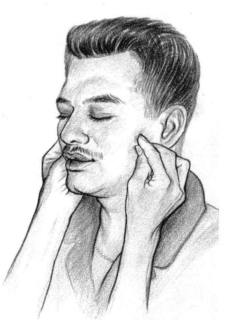

Throat

Gently place your hands on or around the person's throat. There is no need to worry about doing it wrong.

Carpal Tunnel Syndrome and Repetitive Strain Injuries

Carpal Tunnel syndrome may be caused by problems in the wrist, elbow, shoulder, neck, or even lower back, knee, or foot. In most cases you can help speed recovery by working on the wrist, elbow, shoulder, and neck.

Be sure to do the following:

- Run energy directly into the wrist joints. See that the person's hand is in a comfortable upright position as illustrated here.

- Run energy into the area of the seventh cervical and the first thoracic vertebra. (see p. 142)

- If there is pain in the lower back, be sure to run energy there as well.

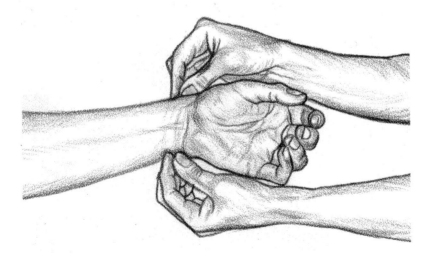

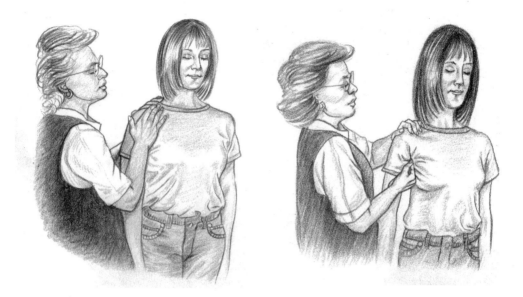

Shoulder Problems

- Run energy directly into the place that hurts. Be sure to ask the person you are working on to make sure that your hands are sandwiching the right position.

- In addition, try running energy from under the armpit and into the shoulder as illustrated.

- If these moves were not successful, try working on the sutures, the occipital ridge, the neck, the lower back, the hips, and then go back to the shoulder.

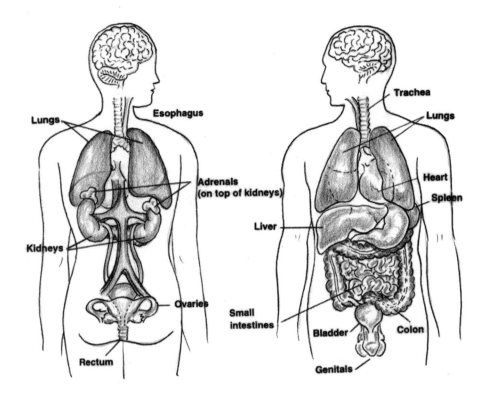

Lungs
Esophagus
Adrenals
(on top of kidneys)
Kidneys
Ovaries
Rectum

Trachea
Lungs
Heart
Spleen
Liver
Small
intestines
Bladder
Colon
Genitals

Organs

Sandwiching works well with most of the organs of the body. You simply have one hand on each side of the body so that the energy will flow between your hands. Keep a dialogue going to find out about sensations your client is having during a session. This information can lead you to work on places that may not have occurred to you.

Simply running energy into the heart can improve blood pressure, heart arrhythmia, and palpitations.

When running energy into the kidneys and adrenals, it works best to work directly over the organs. This approach works well for other organs or parts of the body that are close to the surface, such as the eyes, throat, or bladder.

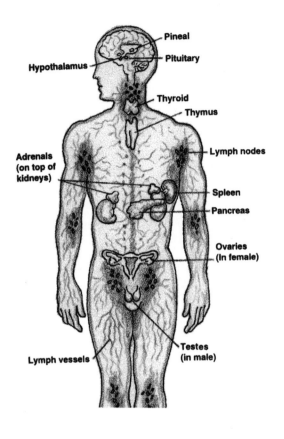

Pineal
Pituitary
Hypothalamus
Thyroid
Thymus
Lymph nodes
Adrenals (on top of kidneys)
Spleen
Pancreas
Ovaries (In female)
Testes (in male)
Lymph vessels

Immune System

You can use the energy to help rebuild or heal the immune system.

- Run energy into the endocrine glands, which include the pineal, pituitary, thyroid, thymus, adrenals, overies and testis.

- Run energy into the lymphatic system, located primarily around the neck, armpits, chest, breasts, stomach, and inner thighs.

- Run energy into major organs – heart, lungs, liver, and kidneys.

- Run the energy anywhere the client is experiencing pains.

With these few simple guidelines, you can do incredible healing work on your family, friends, and those fortunate enough to be near.

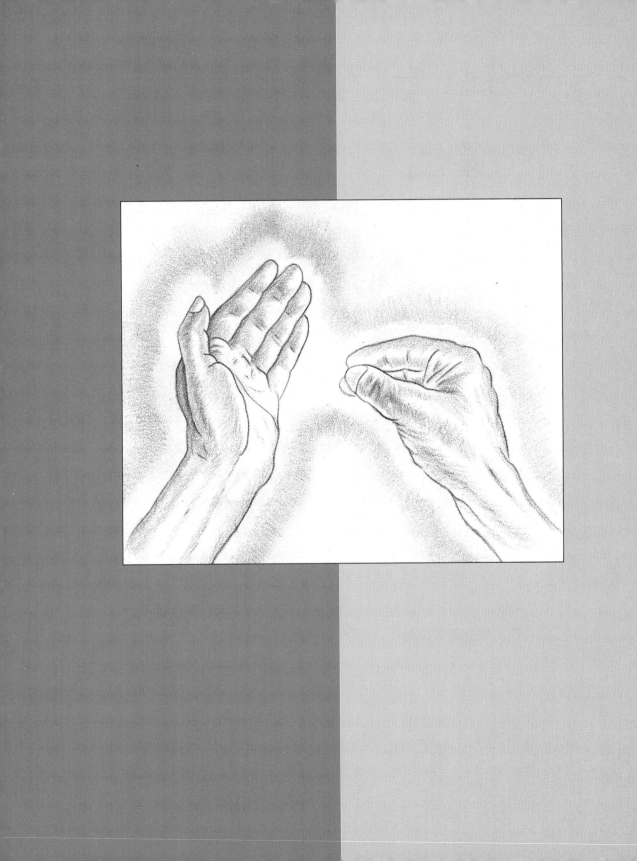

Chapter 10

Self-Healing

The heart of healing is the heart.

Running Energy on Yourself

Giving a session to yourself can be quite wonderful. Having said that, I think it only fair to say that running energy into yourself is usually not as powerful as receiving a session from someone else. Since we are already accustomed to the vibration of our own energy, running our own energy back into ourselves is seldom as spectacular as receiving the energy from another person. A friend of mine to say that, "Healing yourself with energy is a little bit like sex. You can do it on yourself, but it is just not the same."

Receiving love from another person is not predictable or controllable. This is true both energetically and emotionally. I believe that there are many varieties of love – many flavors, if you will. Each person will express their own unique combinations of these qualities. Some people may express their love vibrationally as nurturing, compassion, courage, commitment, trustworthiness, empathy, honesty, vulnerability, intimacy, providing safety, and so on. There are so many delicious flavors of love that just don't fit into a little four-letter word. Perhaps your self-healing needs a flavor of love that you are not accustomed to providing.

There are some conditions I have been able to treat well when running the energy on myself, and others where I was ineffective. For example, while I have been successful working on my eyesight and injuries, I have been unable to adjust the position of my skeletal structure. Be aware that each person is different, and my strengths and weaknesses may certainly not be yours.

A few years ago, I noticed that the moon was becoming blurrier and blurrier when I would look at it, and I wondered why the astronomers were not saying anything about it. I also had to hold books further and further away when I was reading. When I started running energy into my eyes (about five to ten minutes twice a day), I could feel a deep burning sensation, which continued for the first two weeks. About a month after I had begun doing this each day, I walked outside one night and looked at the full moon. It was completely in focus with no blurred edges. It took considerably longer to affect my eyes enough so that I could comfortably read when holding the page closer to me.

Perhaps it is just human nature, but I have tended to get lazy about working on my own eyes. When I practice regularly, I can read from about ten or eleven inches away, and when I stop practicing, after a couple of months, I find myself reading from thirteen or fourteen inches away. Then when I begin again, it only takes a few days to bring my vision back.

About a year ago, I had some oral surgery. By the time I left the dentist's office, the left side of my face was beginning to swell considerably. Behind his office, I sat looking at a river and started running energy into my cheek over where the surgery had been. I spent about an hour and was able to bring the inflammation down about 90 percent. My next appointment was to see my taxman. (This is what I call a good day.) He could not believe that I had just had surgery for a root canal, since I was in no pain and had almost no inflammation. The only time I felt any pain was when I got home. I had just stepped out of my car, and I felt a sudden and intense pain. This pain lasted only a split second and was gone as soon as I put my hand back on my cheek. I spent much of the day with at least one hand touching my cheek. On the three occasions that the dentist operated on that tooth, I needed no pain medication and only occasionally did I feel any hint of pain. This discomfort immediately subsided when I started running the energy.

I remember on another occasion, some friends were helping me move. When I stood up after suddenly lifting a box, I soundly banged the top of my head on a wooden post. This caused me to fall to my knees and "see stars." My immediate inclination was to rub the top of my head, but instead, I forced myself to touch the spot gently with my fingertips and started running energy. After about two minutes, the pain was gone and I went back to work. After about twenty minutes I started wondering if I were going to have one of those bumps on top of my head like those cartoon characters. Very carefully I touched the top of my head and felt no pain. I started pressing harder and harder but could find no indication that I had ever injured myself.

And just so you know that I'm not the only one who can do this, one of my students was slicing vegetables when her knife slipped, and she cut her finger to the bone. She grabbed the finger with her other hand and immediately started running energy into the finger. Within a few minutes the pain and bleeding had stopped. The pain did not return, and she did not need stitches or any other treatment.

It seems that recent injuries may be somewhat easier to self-treat than systemic conditions, since your body has not vibrationally identified with the problem yet.

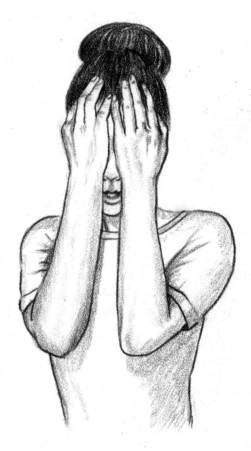

As I was thinking about which of numerous other examples of self-healing to write about, I happened to receive a letter from a friend. She wrote, "By the way, I'm really using Quantum-Touch these days. I slipped in dance class and bruised my knee with a bump the size of a large fried egg. I ran energy in it after class and within hours, it is only slightly pink now, with almost no swelling, and is very minimal in size. Hey, it works!"

Guidelines for Self-Healing Sessions

- Practice running energy into yourself regularly and often. Self-healing may require many sessions, so when you practice full body sweeps and running energy, it can be a good idea to run energy into yourself. You can practice while watching TV or movies, or even reading a book. This may be a one-handed session unless you find a special way of holding the book.

- Sandwich any part of your body that you can reach comfortably, and place your hands directly over those places that you cannot sandwich. For example, it would be hard to sandwich your own heart between your hands, so place both hands over your heart.

- If you are working on an inaccessible place, like the middle of the back, you can use distant healing techniques as described in chapter 12.

- To make sessions as strong as possible, pump the breath by exaggerating the breathing techniques. If you lie down, you can do the fire breath for much longer periods without feeling dizzy. In this way, you can alter your vibration more profoundly and be more effective. (People with certain heart conditions may not be able to do this safely. If you are unsure, check with your physician.)

- This can be a great time to try combinations of techniques; that is, you can do more than one technique at the same time. For example, you could be doing toning and the amplified resonance technique (chapter 12) while you work on yourself.

- Be patient. Many people will gladly spend forty or sixty minutes when working on a friend, but can hardly find five or ten minutes to work on themselves.

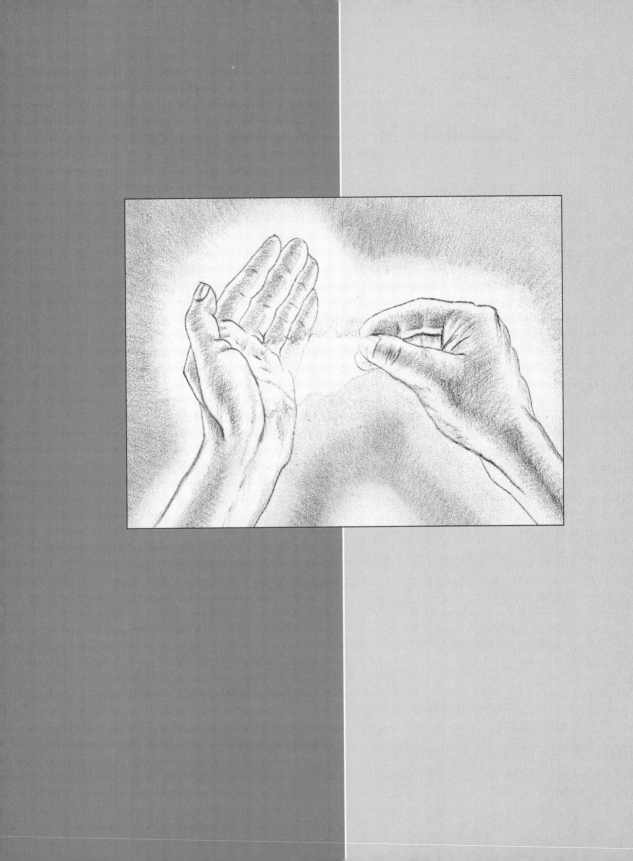

Chapter 11

Healing Animals

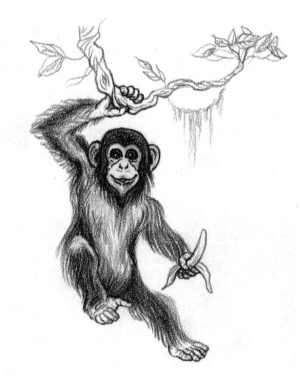

"Monkeys are my favorite people."

– Unknown

Working with animals can be a wondrous joy, since their love is so available and their affection is so generously given. Our pets and other animals do not judge us for our age, weight, race, or lifestyle. What's more, they have no prejudices favoring Western allopathic medicine – they simply respond to love.

Quantum-Touch has worked wonderfully well on all sorts of animals: dogs, cats, horses, mice, turtles, even bunny rabbits. It seems to make no difference. Everybody seems to like animal stories, so I'll tell you a few.

When I arrived in Maine to teach a class last year, I stayed at Billie's home. As she had advertised, she had ten cats, all longhaired Maine coons. In my conversations with Billie, I had learned that Julius (who has a technique named after him in chapter 5), Billie's favorite cat, had been very ill for a couple of months. She had taken the cat to the veterinarian a few times, but they could not help him or even figure out what his problem was. As soon as I got to her home I saw cats everywhere, but off to the side was one cat whose fur was all scruffy, and he looked as if he had passed out on the arm of the couch. I immediately knew that I had found Julius.

I put my bags down and walked straight over to him, and introduced myself (in cat language, this meant letting the cat sniff my hand). Julius seemed terribly limp and weak, his fur was slightly damp, and he appeared to hardly have the strength to lift his head. I started to run energy into his abdomen and within a minute or two, I realized that I was dealing with what I call the "blocked pattern" of energy as described in chapter 3. As I ran energy in for about five minutes, the vibration was only starting to get a bit stronger. At that point, I called Billie and Heather and asked them to help me. Heather and Billie are both accomplished Quantum-Touch practitioners, and group sessions are generally much easier and faster.

The three of us ran energy for another ten minutes, and Julius got up to stretch and then jumped down to the floor. I didn't think much of the session at the time. A couple minutes later I had found a cat toy consisting of a stick with a string and a ball at the end of the string. As I dragged the ball around the floor, I was surrounded by a circle of cats that were politely waiting for the ball to get to them before they would take a good swipe at it.

When Julius saw the game, he did something that Billie said she had never seen him do. He started leaping a couple of feet, straight up in the air almost like a gazelle. He did this three or four times as if he were bouncing towards the game. When he got there, he completely took over as he repeatedly jumped across the entire circle to get to the ball. A few minutes later, Billie opened her door and Julius was the first one outside.

Julius has had no more health problems since that single session. When I returned about seven months later to teach another Quantum-Touch class, I had the opportunity to spend time with him again. He seemed to recognize me and was extremely affectionate. I decided to run energy into him to see what would happen this time. He just loved it and got more and more excited. This time, he grabbed my hand and was licking and biting and scratching me in a playful manner that was beginning to hurt a bit. After a few seconds of this, Julius looked at me and saw I was not enjoying this and immediately stopped biting. He got up and walked away.

An hour later, Billie told me that Julius had done something else that he had never done before – he had caught a bird. It seems that both sessions really brought out the kitty cat's "inner tiger." I have heard similar stories about cats wanting to go into hunting mode after a good Quantum-Touch session.

On another occasion, a friend had a dog (a Newfoundland) that had problems with its sacroiliac. The dog could not walk, and they had to take it to a veterinarian in an ambulance. The vet said that in most cases like this one, the dog has to be put to sleep. When I saw the dog, he was home again and unable to walk. After two sessions over a two-day period, the dog was walking again with no problems.

You may recall in the first chapter how I ran energy into a frightened young bunny and it reacted by rolling onto its back and stretching out as far as it could. My friend Henri has had very similar results with her turtle. He's an 8-inch-long African Sideneck, and by nature extremely shelter-conscious. In the wild, his habitat would be at the water's edge, near overhanging ferns, or burrowing into tight spaces to escape predators. He avoids any kind of exposure, and never basks in the sun. Henri writes, "When I run energy into him, I hold him in my lap. One hand cups his upper shell, the other is underneath. Within seconds, he closes his eyes. As I continue to run energy, he relaxes totally, extending his neck forward, his arms and legs spread-eagle. We can stay like this for minutes or hours."

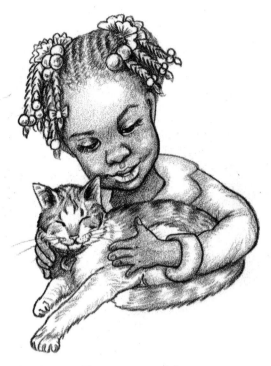

I'll tell you one more story to whet your appetite for doing sessions on animals. A friend asked me to do Quantum-Touch work on her horse. I'm not one of those people who spends time with horses, but I thought I would enjoy the new experience. On a sunny afternoon, I was running energy into the horse's back, and she said that I was "putting the horse to sleep." "I hope you don't mean in the veterinary sense," I told her. She said, "No, you are actually putting the horse to sleep." "How can you tell?" I asked. "Just look at his eyes," she replied. I looked at her horse's eyes and saw that they were drooping and closing, while her lower lip was hanging and trembling. A moment later the horse's head just dropped, like a person who falls asleep sitting up. The horse was awake again and now rested his head on a metal rail by its stall. As I continued giving the horse energy, its head slipped off the metal railing three more times.

Just as in my human patients, I never know what the energy is doing. I just trust that something wonderful is happening.

Guidelines for Working with Animals

- Be sure to sandwich or run energy directly into any area that you think needs healing. A diagnosis from a veterinarian may help you pinpoint the problem.

- Be sure to keep your breathing techniques going the whole time you work.

- Since the animal can't talk, pay close attention to the sensations in your hands as described in chapter 3. This will help you to know how long to keep your hands in any one place.

- Realize that you are not going to do it "wrong." Energy finds its way to where it needs to go and does what needs to be done.

- Give a series of sessions if necessary.

- When you are brushing your animal's hair, try running energy into them at the same time. This works with any kind of petting motion, whether it's scratching behind their ears or rubbing their tummy.

- Try running energy into them before or while giving them a bath. For a special treat, energize the bath water as well (see chapter 15). This works especially well if baths are not on your animal's list of fun things to experience.

- You can also run energy into their food and water, as well as your own (see chapter 15). For animals primarily eating canned food, it really increases the energetic signature of their food.

I'm sure you will be quite surprised and delighted by the results of your work.

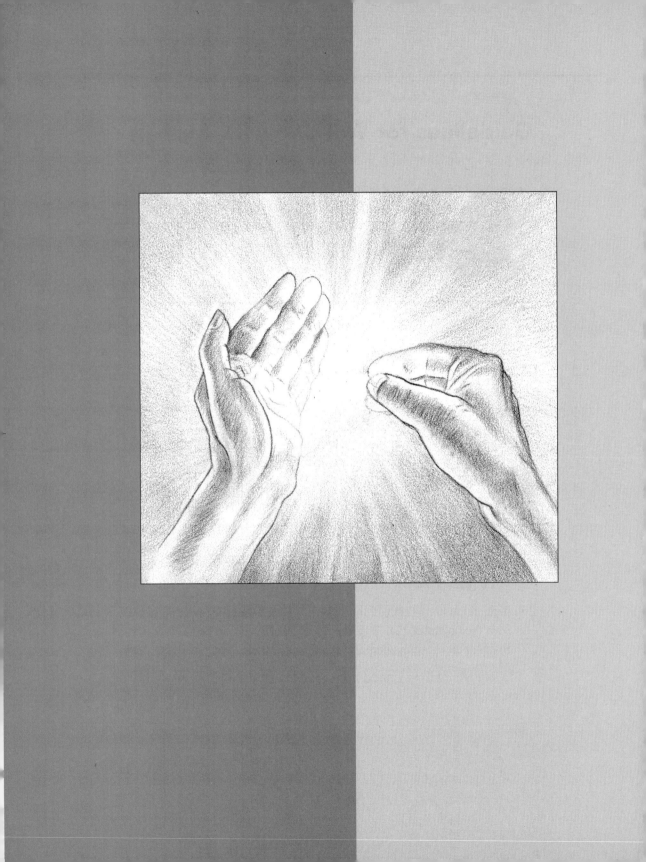

Chapter 12

Distant Healing

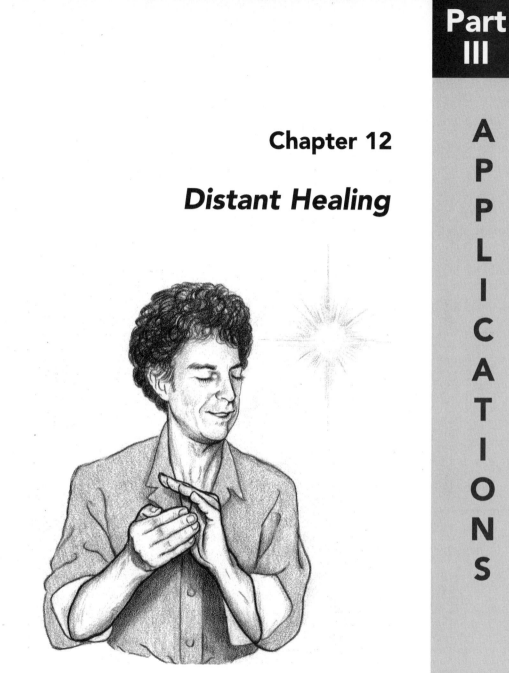

*Infinitely faster than the speed of light, our compassion
and our prayers move at the velocity of love
It's instantaneous!*

On Being Connected

I believe that we are all far more connected to one another than the consensus would have us believe. On a personal level, the well-being of family and friends is often much more important to us than we may acknowledge daily. A sudden loss can bring this point into sharp focus. Although many people become indifferent or deadened by the media's drone of bad news, sometimes the story of the loss of a child or leader whom we have never met touches us profoundly. Economically we see that problems on one continent may immediately impact all world markets. Globally, we have only one big ocean and all share the same water, the same air, and the same earth. Our lives and fate are inextricably linked. What you may not be aware of is that even the very smallest of particles are linked in a surprisingly profound manner.

Numerous books have been written about the strange and almost magical world of quantum physics. In Gary Zukav's fine book, *The Dancing Wu Li Masters*, he writes:

> Bell's theorem is a mathematical construct which, as such, is indecipherable to the nonmathematician. Its implications however, could affect profoundly our basic world view. Some physicists are convinced that it is the most important single work, perhaps, in the history of physics. One of the implications of Bell's theorem is that, at a deep and fundamental level, the "separate parts" of the universe are connected in an intimate and immediate way... Suppose that we have what physicists call a two-particle system of zero spin. This means that the spin of each of the particles in the system cancels the other. If one of the particles in such a system has a spin up, the other particle has a spin down. If the first particle has a spin right, the second particle has a spin left. No matter how the particles are oriented, their spins are always equal and opposite.

Many quantum physicists have become upset as they have pondered how paired photons, traveling away from each other at the speed of light, are able to somehow respond to one another instantaneously, infinitely faster than the speed of light.

If these two particles are sent in opposite directions, no matter how far apart they may become, they are still linked. They could be thousands of light years away from one another, but if one of the particles goes through a magnetic device that changes its spin, say from up to down, the other particle, regardless of distance, will instantaneously and spontaneously change its spin from down to up. I believe that the impact of our love travels in a similar sort of fashion.

I have often thought about our interconnectedness in an intellectual or spiritual sense, but the actual sense of being physically linked to one another was brought home to me in a powerful and personal way when I visited Dr. C. Norman Shealy, M.D., Ph.D. at his clinic in Springfield, Missouri. After demonstrating how Quantum-Touch affects posture and showing him how effective it is in treating some of his most difficult chronic pain patients, Dr. Shealy decided to see how Quantum-Touch might affect brain wave patterns at a distance. This was something that I had never tried, and to be honest, I was not at all confident about the outcome.

Dr. Shealy asked an elderly gentleman to lie down for an hour to have his brainwaves mapped out. The man had not been told that I would be trying to do a distant healing session on him. When I use the word "distant," I mean that there is no physical contact being made between the practitioner and client. In this case, I was only about twelve feet away, but based on my experience and that of others, it would not have mattered if I were twelve miles or twelve thousand miles away. For thirty minutes, we monitored the man's brainwaves and used that information as a baseline. At this point, one of Norm's assistants tapped me on the shoulder as a signal to start doing distant healing. For the next thirty minutes I ran the energy and when I was finished, we continued monitoring his brainwaves for another five minutes to see if stopping had an effect.

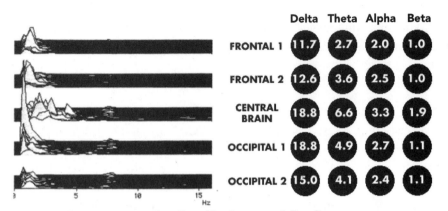

	Delta	Theta	Alpha	Beta
FRONTAL 1	11.7	2.7	2.0	1.0
FRONTAL 2	12.6	3.6	2.5	1.0
CENTRAL BRAIN	18.8	6.6	3.3	1.9
OCCIPITAL 1	18.8	4.9	2.7	1.1
OCCIPITAL 2	15.0	4.1	2.4	1.1

The data above represents a baseline of brainwave activity after the subject had been resting for thirty minutes.

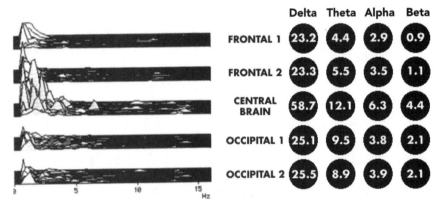

	Delta	Theta	Alpha	Beta
FRONTAL 1	23.2	4.4	2.9	0.9
FRONTAL 2	23.3	5.5	3.5	1.1
CENTRAL BRAIN	58.7	12.1	6.3	4.4
OCCIPITAL 1	25.1	9.5	3.8	2.1
OCCIPITAL 2	25.5	8.9	3.9	2.1

Five munutes after the distant healing had begun. Note the significant increase of delta activity.

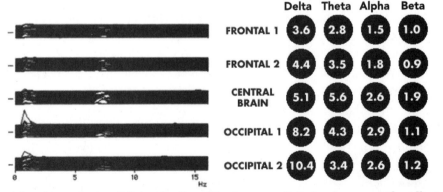

	Delta	Theta	Alpha	Beta
FRONTAL 1	3.6	2.8	1.5	1.0
FRONTAL 2	4.4	3.5	1.8	0.9
CENTRAL BRAIN	5.1	5.6	2.6	1.9
OCCIPITAL 1	8.2	4.3	2.9	1.1
OCCIPITAL 2	10.4	3.4	2.6	1.2

After thirty minutes of distant healing all brainwave activity has become profoundly quiet.

The results surprised me a great deal. In the first five minutes after I started running energy, the man's delta brain wave activity increased profoundly. In the left and right frontal parts of his brain, delta waves jumped from 11.7 and 12.6 respectively, to 23.2 and 23.3. The midbrain readout jumped from 18.8 to 58.7, and occipital readouts went up from 18.8 and 15.0 to 25.0 and 26.3. By the end of the session, his frontal delta readouts had dropped to an amazing 3.6 and 4.4, his midbrain was down to 5.1, and the occipital readings became 8.2 and 10.4, respectively. Dr. Shealy told me that in thirty years of looking at brain waves, he had never seen such a quiet pattern. He added that if he had not known better and had only seen the last readout of brain activity, he might have thought the man was brain-dead. I find this comment especially interesting, coming from an former neurosurgeon.

In the weeks that followed that experience, I realized that I had been shaken again by the profundity of the work. Deep inside, I had not believed that my thoughts could have had so much impact, but they clearly did. As I contemplated what had happened, it occurred to me that the distant healing work demonstrates how connected we all are to one another and gave me another little taste of just how powerful our love is.

When we are touching someone during a session, we are clearly assisting to change the vibration of the tissue in a very direct way. This is what I have come to call "local healing" because of the proximity of the practitioner to the client. In "nonlocal healing," the practitioner may be five or ten feet away, or possibly on the moon, and the impact would be just as strong, since the field is created by thought.

One of the ways that distant healing differs from local healing is that the field created in the distant work does not easily move the structure. That is, bones do not simultaneously adjust as they do from the local healings. Given that that is the case, it appears that the distant healing work sets up a different sort of field than the local healing. It occurred to me that by holding the distant field and the local field at once, we could set up a synergy of vibration not unlike having two people working together. The results are quite profound and gratifying.

When I teach my Quantum-Touch classes, I lead groups to do a distant healing on all the people who are in the room. The experience is quite immediate and dramatic, as almost everyone can clearly feel the energy. Like anything else, distant healing work seems to have its strengths and its limitations.

Here are just a couple of examples to give you a taste of how distant healing can work.

One of my students named John had told me about his aunt who had a tumor. He was very concerned about her. At exactly seven o'clock that evening John set out to send her some energy. He focused deeply, did the breathing techniques, and continued for a full thirty minutes. A little after eight, he called her on the phone and started chatting about things: how is your husband, how are the kids, what's happening. . . after about fifteen minutes John asked her how her health was, particularly her tumor. Suddenly her voice became all excited and animated, saying that it has been the most amazing thing, at exactly seven p.m., she could feel "all this energy going into the tumor," and she told him that it felt like it was draining and getting smaller. He asked her how long that continued, and she said that it had been for exactly thirty minutes, but now it was feeling all warm and wonderful, and she was enthusiastic about her potential to be healed. He said that he didn't want to tell her what he had been doing because he didn't think that she would understand. Apparently she could appreciate the love, if not the explanation.

I was talking with my friend Lauri over the phone one evening, and she told me that she was having a severe allergy attack and was having some distressing back pain. Having been trained as a registered nurse, Lauri was preparing to medicate herself, but was feeling reluctant because she knew that the medication would "knock her out" for a couple of days so that she could not function effectively. I invited her to come over and let me work on her, but she said it was too late and she was not feeling well enough to drive. "Then let me do some distant healing," I suggested. She was adamant about taking her medication and I protested. We finally negotiated that if she were not feeling better after one hour she would go ahead and take her medication. I started to run the energy, and after twenty-five minutes, my phone rang. She called to say that not only had all her allergy symptoms cleared out, but her back pain had disappeared as well.

Guidelines for Doing Distant Healing

- **Get permission.** It is always a good idea to get permission to do distant healing. If for one reason or another you cannot get permission, simply ask that the energy be used for the highest good, and send it to the person. Sending the energy for the highest good is a great thing to do anyway.

- **Connect with the person being healed.** Whether you are sending energy to a person, animal, or plant, you need to know to whom the energy will go. If you don't know the subject personally, it can really help to have a photo to help you focus and direct the energy.

- **Connect with your spirituality**. This is useful for those who have an inclination to do so. Asking for help can only improve the work.

- **Use a surrogate object to help you focus.** Admittedly, it takes more concentration to stay focused when you are doing distant healing. You can't just leave your hands on the person and focus on your breathing; you need to keep intending that the energy go where you are sending it. For these reasons, many people like to hold an object such as a teddy bear, pillow, or blanket to give them a physical point of focus. It isn't necessary to use a surrogate, but it is an option if you choose to use it.

- **Bring your attention to the place that needs the energy and imagine that it is between your hands.** You can imagine and see that the very place you are sending the energy is right between your hands. Since you are using your imagination, you can be working directly on organs or other tissue. The key here is not only to bring your attention to the place you wish to send the energy, but to keep your attention there while you run the energy.

- **Use the breathing and run the energy.** As in all Quantum-Touch work, keep the breathing going and powerfully run the energy out your hands.

- **Combine different techniques.** Distant healing can be a great opportunity to experiment and combine any of the various techniques during the session.

- **Take your time.** Distant healing sessions may last thirty, forty-five, or sixty minutes. This can take a lot of commitment on the part of the practitioner.

- **Don't be attached to outcome.** As in other Quantum-Touch work, it is important to keep in mind that you are simply holding a resonance and that they are responsible to do the healing.

It is so wonderful to realize that our love really does have impact and can be felt by those people we wish to send it to. Now when I might use the phrase, "Send her my love," I suddenly realize, "Hey, I can also do it myself!"

The Amplified Resonance Technique

The amplified resonance technique is a hands-on technique that also employs skills of distant healing, so I have placed it in this chapter. This technique is extremely powerful and has become one of my favorite approaches to running the energy. The AR technique, as we have come to call it, does require a good deal of skill and concentration since you are doing two things at once.

1. Place your hands on the client as you would normally do and start running the energy.

2. While you are running the energy out your hands, use your mind to "enter into" the tissue being treated. With each breath hold your mind inside the tissue you are working on and stay there while you are simultaneously running the energy out of your hands.

When I say to use your mind to enter the tissue, I am suggesting that you hold your point of attention inside the part of their body that you are working on. You don't have to have any particular visualization about what is going on in the tissue you are working on; you need only use your intention to keep your awareness there. If you want to, you can imagine that the part of the body you are sending your attention to is lit up with light. Another possibility is to imagine that you are bringing a ball of energy that is physically inside the area you are working on and get it spinning. The main point is that you keep your attention trained on that place. With your mind, you are running the energy into their body, and while you keep the breathing going, you are also running the energy out of your hands.

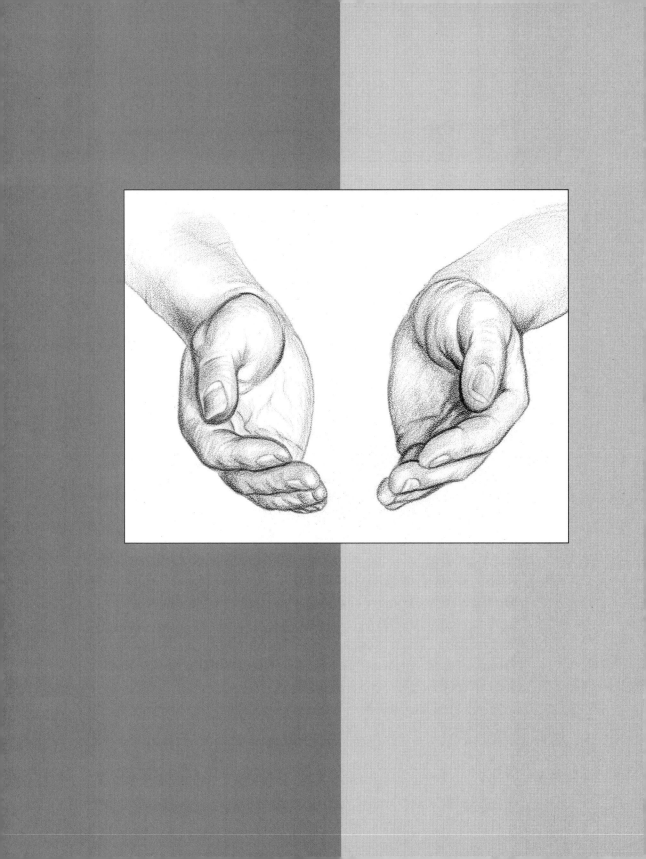

Chapter 13

Emotional Healing

*Beneath the murky waters of unwanted and
disowned emotion lie the vast and hidden
treasures of who we truly are.*

Emotions and the Healing Process

Five of us were giving a group session to Helen. She had been one of Dr. Norman Shealy's most difficult chronic pain patients who had not responded to any traditional or alternative therapy. About twenty minutes into the session, she was becoming extremely distressed. When we asked her what the matter was, she said, "There are emotions coming up that I don't want to feel and I'm afraid that if I feel these emotions, they are so dark, I'm scared that I'll never be okay again." It was in August of 1998, and I was showing Dr. Shealy and his staff how effective Quantum-Touch was at treating chronic pain patients. At that moment, Helen was receiving a Quantum-Touch session by me, Dr. Shealy, and three of his staff. In the following minutes the level of her distress continued to increase, and Dr. Shealy talked with her and the rest of us kept up the breathing.

In the kindest and most nurturing way, Dr. Shealy encouraged Helen to let herself feel the emotions that were coming up. "No, no, no," she protested, "if I let myself feel these emotions, I'll be stuck in those feelings for the rest of my life." After a few minutes of compassionate and gentle persuasion, Dr. Shealy assisted her to feel safe enough to let the emotions begin to come out. She then went through an intense wave of crying that lasted for about five minutes, and soon after that, she started to feel quite wonderful. Another fifteen minutes into the session, and she started feeling a whole new wave of sadness. Again, she protested, if she let herself feel the emotions, she would be stuck there forever. Dr. Shealy once again reassured her that this was not the case and that she would be okay. Feeling safer, she then let the next wave of emotions surge through her. This wave of grief rose even more intensely than before. After some minutes of tears, joy once again filled the space where the pain had been.

By the end of the session, she reported that about 70 percent of her physical pain had been relieved. This was pain that for ten years had not responded to any traditional or alternative therapy that was attempted. When we asked her what she had experienced emotionally, she said that she had been grieving because she knew that in this life, she would never have a baby. Somehow, by letting herself completely feel the intensity of these emotions, much of her physical pain had lifted off as well. Helen even went on to say how she could now be excited about her future and accept herself as a creative and successful person without a child to raise.

Emotions rising up during Quantum-Touch sessions are not uncommon. *I find it fascinating how the specific emotions that bring on cathartic experiences seem to consistently be the emotions that had been suppressed, oppressed, or repressed. So often, the act of courageously allowing these emotions to be fully experienced is exactly what is necessary for relieving or transforming physical conditions.* I'm convinced that the biggest human blockage is the unwillingness to fully experience the intensity of our emotions.

For most people, the expression of anger is especially difficult and frightening. It is often not easy to express a variety of other emotions such as hurt, humiliation, shame, dread, rage, and hate. Sadly, the positive emotions become suppressed as well. Many people will live a painful life filled with shame, rage, and dread, and thus avoid feeling something really scary, like the wondrous depth of their own magnificence.

When you shine light upon a shadow, it disappears.

It is well beyond the scope of this book to deal with the primary issues of emotional causation. Here are some approaches you can use in your Quantum-Touch sessions.

Guidelines for Working with Emotions that Arise During a Session

- **Trust the process**. Admittedly, it can be distressing watching someone go through intense emotions. The most important thing that I have relied on over the years is to simply trust the process. I just keep running the energy until things naturally work themselves out. The worst thing to do would be to get scared and stop the session. It is best to give kind reassurance to your client that it is okay to feel what he or she is feeling and to keep breathing and running the energy.

- **Grounding**. Maintain sensations inside your body as I have described in chapter 3. This will help you stay grounded and in a better place to help. (Grounding is described in chapter 4)

- **Keep breathing**. Keep breathing and encourage your friend to breathe too. This can accelerate the process and protect those people who tend to take on the other person's symptoms or emotions.

- **Run energy into the part of their body where they are feeling the emotions**. This is a wonderful technique that can powerfully assist your friend to find their emotional balance and move through the feelings that arise. Sandwich the area front and back so they feel cradled by your hands. If they are sitting up, you might have them lean forward as you support their weight. (I know a number of psychotherapists who use this approach to help their patients become centered and more responsibly process emotions.)

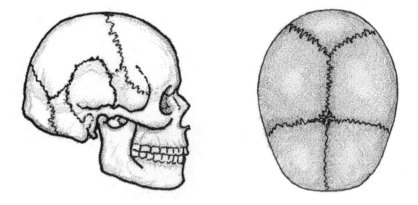

- **Run energy into the sutures and the brain.** The sutures are the spaces where cranial bones connect to one another. Emotional imbalances can cause the sutures to move out of alignment. Spending five or fifteen minutes running energy into the sutures can be very helpful for assisting people to find their own emotional balance. Bob Rasmusson liked to tell the story of a woman who was grieving uncontrollably when her baby died. After running energy into her sutures, it wasn't that she was done grieving, but she could also feel grateful for having known the child.

- **Run energy into the chakras.** Running energy into each chakra is a great way to balance emotions and may assist in the release of the emotions as well. You can run energy into each of their chakras, and give extra attention to the chakras closest to the part of their body where they are feeling the emotions most profoundly. Sandwiching the chakra points front and back can work very well.

In most cases, it would be awkward or embarrassing to touch people over their first and second chakras. An alternative to placing the hands on the perineum, which is between the anus and the genitals, is to contact a point about an inch below the navel. This point reflexes to the first chakra. The other hand can touch the tailbone, so together they make a nice contact with the first chakra. The second chakra can be contacted by placing fingertips on the very top of the pubic bone. If this is too threatening to your friend or client, you can run energy into the inside and outside of the heels. If you press lightly into the sides of the heels, you will likely find tender points. These are great places to run the energy.

- **Run energy into the occipital ridge**. This can help to break up old thought and emotional patterns and can sometimes help with addictions.

- **Use distant healing**. Distant healing can be useful when treating psychotherapy patients where actually touching them is not therapeutic, is contraindicated, or not physically possible.

I think it is important to remember that the goal of working with people's emotions is not to heal their emotions, but to assist them energetically to release what needs releasing or let them naturally come into their own emotional balance. Like water seeking its own level, the emotional body seeks to find balance. It is not your job to fix anyone, and given the opportunity, people will naturally heal themselves.

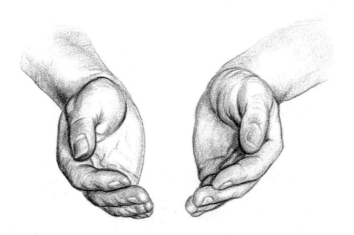

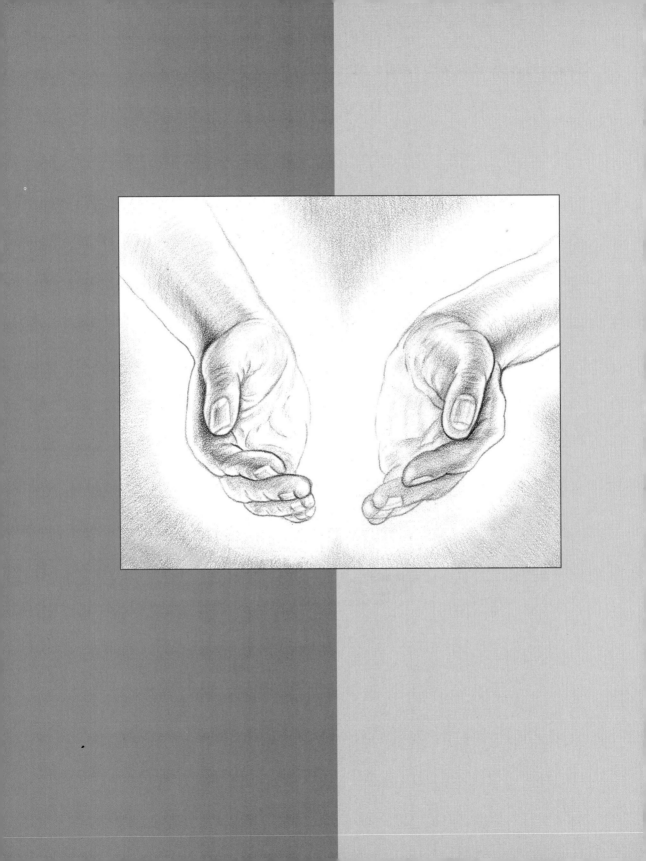

Chapter 14

Fun Stuff

"Life is a gift, and ours is but to learn to receive it."
– Lazaris

When I was a child, I remember daydreaming in school about how great it would be to invent or to discover something truly wonderful. My next thought was more discouraging: so many great things had already been invented, and who was I to ever come up with anything anyway?

One of the aspects of Quantum-Touch that thoroughly delights me is that just about anyone who decides to experiment and play with the life-force energy can discover and invent new applications or techniques. This experimentation can be hardly more than playful fun, yet quite valuable things can be discovered and learned.

I have divided up this chapter into three sections: "Fun with Inanimate Objects," "Fun with Food," and "Fun with People." I like to think of creativity and exploration as fun, yet I take my fun seriously. Serendipitous discoveries often lead to many of the most important breakthroughs. So I encourage you to play with these suggestions, have fun, and make your own discoveries, and when you have learned something new, write to us and tell us what you have found. We expect to come out with a newsletter from time to time to share stories, discoveries, insights, and of course, news. So if you are ready, let's play.

Fun with Inanimate Objects

Belts and Gloves

Take an ordinary leather belt and gently hold it over a friend's temples like a headband. Lightly place your thumb, index finger, and ring fingers of each hand (the tripod position) on the belt, directly over your friend's temples, and run energy into the belt for about two minutes. After you have done this, now run the energy directly into your friend's temples without the belt around their forehead. I've tried this little test many times and have seen that people who are able to feel the energy when they are touched are not able to feel it when energy is being run through the belt.

One intriguing and extremely interesting property of leather is that it seems to only absorb life-force energy, and doesn't let it go. No matter how much energy you run into a common leather belt, in my experience, you will not be able to "fill it with energy." No matter how long you

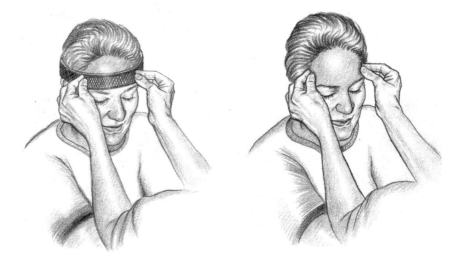

spend running the energy into leather, the leather never gets to the point where the energy starts to pass through or to radiate out the other side.

This small and seemingly unimportant piece of information may prove to be extremely valuable when double-blind tests are conducted. Simply having non-trained practitioners wearing thin leather gloves will effectively block out the healing properties of the ambient life-force. The benefit of the "gloved sessions" would, therefore, be for testing the placebo effect.

We also tested rubber gloves in the same manner as leather belts and found that only a fraction of the energy passes through the gloves. Although it is hard to be exact, the consensus is that approximately one third of the energy is able to penetrate the glove. I should also mention, while I'm on the subject, that thick nylon and polyester are also able to block the energy as well as leather. I'm not sure if this has any health implications to the wearer of heavy nylon, polyester, or leather, but I believe that it is worth noting.

Since leather was once alive, perhaps it is absorbing the energy as a very ineffective sort of healing. This may sound somewhat far-fetched, but when you read about my experience with a guitar, you may reconsider.

Fun with <u>Your</u> Expensive Guitar or Stradivarius

I own a 35-year-old nylon string guitar that has an excellent, clear, and bright sound. One day I had the clever idea of running energy into the wood of my guitar. As you may have gathered by now, I like trying new things. Perhaps this sounds a little crazy, but I've been accused of worse.

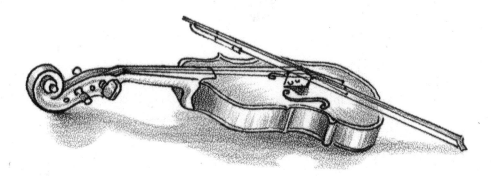

As I ran the energy for about six or eight minutes, I could not feel any energy connection; that is to say, it seemed that the wood was not responding to the energy. This is what I referred to previously as the "blocked pattern". Then, gradually, I was able to start feeling an energy field slowly increasing between my hands and the wood. By the end of about fifty minutes, I had run energy into the entire top and back of my guitar. I was so excited to play my guitar and to see how great it would sound. I turned the guitar over and played a chord. Instead of hearing that bright and clear sound, it sounded like a distinct thud, as if the guitar were filled with water. No matter what I played, it sounded like I was playing on a $20 guitar with 10-year-old strings.

My first reaction was to be quite excited and elated to think that I could actually cause so much effect on the resonance of the wood. My next reaction was one of denial, that this couldn't possibly be true. I cleaned the guitar, went out and bought new strings, and figured that it must be my imagination. After the new strings were on for three days, I carefully tuned it with my electric tuner and decided that it would surely sound good now, because I must surely have made the whole thing up. The new strings sounded only about 5 percent better than the old strings. My third reaction was one of grief. "Oh my God, I killed my guitar."

After I priced out a new guitar and decided I didn't like that option, as a last resort, I used an old guitar maker's trick. I leaned the guitar against a stereo speaker and kept music playing through the guitar whenever I left the house. After a few months of reverberating the wood, the guitar started to sound pretty good again. I believe that the guitar is at least as good as before I started. It might even be a bit better, but I can't be sure.

As with many discoveries, one is left with far more questions than answers. My best theory is that the energy somehow altered the position of water molecules and thus affected the resonance of the wood, making it sound waterlogged. Perhaps in a way similar to the leather gloves, the energy was trying to bring life back into the wood.

I have one final comment. Please note that the title of this section is, "Fun with Your Expensive Guitar or Stradivarius." The word "your" is placed there quite intentionally; I'm not going to try it again with mine!

Fun with Water and Food

Charging water

If you would like to send life-force energy to every one of your hundred trillion cells, all you have to do is charge water and drink it. Charging water or any other fluid is quite easy to do. Using both hands, simply hold the glass or bottle with your palms or fingertips only, so your left and right hands are not touching each other, and then run energy into the water for a few minutes or longer. This hand position forces the energy to pass into the fluid that is between your hands.

A couple of physicists explained to me that water has the ability to alter its hydrogen bonding and can hold an infinite variety of structures. I believe that Quantum-Touch works on a subatomic level of matter, which could explain how this could be possible.

Water changes its taste when you run energy into it, and the extent of the change will often depend on the source of the water and the extent of the charge. For a few years, I informally charged one of two glasses of water when no one was watching and would hand them to people and ask them to taste each of them and tell me what they noticed. Without any coaching, people keep using the same words to describe the water that had been charged. In the vast majority of cases, people called the water "silkier," "smoother," "softer," "better tasting," "less metallic," "less chlorine taste," and occasionally some have called the charged water "thicker" or even "syrupy."

A few years ago, I was documenting Quantum-Touch sessions on the men's and women's basketball teams at the University of California in Santa Cruz, where an average ten-minute session reduced their pain levels by 50 percent. One evening, two of the women players complained loudly about how awful the tap water tasted. They had filled up their plastic bottles with the water from the drinking fountain and were making ugly faces and disparaging remarks every time they drank from their plastic bottles. I asked one of them to let me see if I could help out. I held a bottle for about two or three minutes and ran energy into it. When I had finished, she took the bottle back and took a drink. "It is not good," she said. She then took a drink from her friend's bottle and made a really ugly face and more disparaging remarks I will not repeat here. Her friend drank from both bottles with the same reactions.

To conduct their own little experiment, they called two more players off the court, and without explaining anything, they held out the two bottles and said, "Taste these bottles of water and tell us what you think." The two women tasted the bottles and had exactly the same reactions as the women who had watched me charge the bottles. They each said that the charged water did not taste good, but when they tasted the uncharged water, they each made ugly faces and added to the highly disparaging remarks.

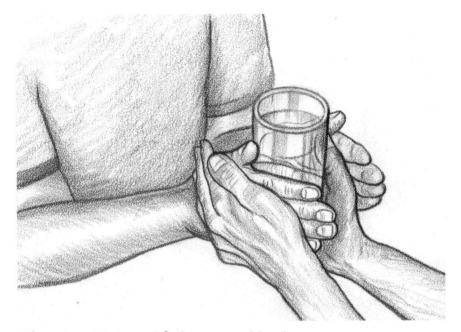

Charging Water with Someone You Love

Here is a nice little variation on charging water. Get a glass of water and have you and a friend charge it together. Use the stacking of hands technique I described previously. When you charge water together, there is a wonderful synergistic effect that is greater than the sum of the parts. When you are done, go ahead and share the water that you charged. This can be a lovely little ritual, blessing, or prayer.

Charging Wine

Charging wine can be a lot of fun. I have found that it is easier to demonstrate charging white wine than red wine. For a long time, people were telling me that the aftertaste was markedly reduced when the white wine was charged, and most people I talked to liked the difference. Out of curiosity one day, I went to a winery and asked the woman who was pouring wine if she would help me understand what people are looking for when they taste wine. She poured different samples and had me notice the bouquet, the complexity, the aftertaste, and so on. I asked her if she would taste wine that I charged and tell me what she thought. At first she refused because she was certain nothing would change. I finally begged her to please humor me and help me get over any delusions I had about altering the taste of wine.

She carefully tasted each of the samples twice, comparing the charged to the uncharged sample. She tasted each a second time to be sure of her findings and then posed a question to me. "Do you realize what you have done? Do you realize what you have done?" "No, please tell me," I asked. "You have destroyed the complexity of this wine, and you have nearly demolished the aftertaste as well." "Is that good?" I asked sheepishly. "NO! It is very, very *bad*!" Just to be sure she really meant this, I teased her a bit, raising my arms up for effect, and said, "If you would like, I could charge all the bottles around here at once." She immediately became loud and adamant, while waving her arms and shouting, "*No, don't do that!*"

Grapefruit Juice

It is fun to run energy into grapefruit juice because it tends to flatten out the stinging aftertaste. Most people like the stinging aftertaste and don't like the charged juice as much, but it is fun to see the difference.

Carbonation

Some children showed me that they can flatten the carbonation of soft drinks, and remove much of the sweet taste by running energy into it. We found that even some adults can do this.

Running Energy into Food or Drinks and Vitamins

Go ahead and charge up your food, drinks, and nutritional supplements. Just hold your hands over your food and run the energy. The field will charge your food. Go ahead and charge up your vitamins too. If you bless your food, you can include this as part of the blessing.

Fun with People

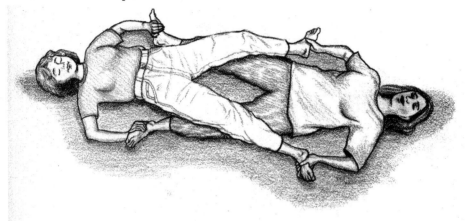

Chakra Charging for Two

This is a lovely healing and balancing technique where both people are simultaneously giving and receiving. Mutual chakra charging can be a marvelous way to share love, to relax, to experience healing, or to drift into wonderful altered states of consciousness.

With a little practice, this technique can become a favorite with couples or friends who wish to explore the possibilities. In order to do this successfully, both people need to know how to run energy and do the chakra work as described in chapters 5 and 6. The more powerfully each of you runs the energy and the longer you do this (as long as it is comfortable), the more successful the outcome will be.

In the position as pictured above, each person spins their own first chakra and runs the energy out their hands into the other person's feet. When both people feel that they have built up a strong charge, they can move on to the second chakra. Continue in this manner through all seven chakras and then work with chakras eight through twelve.

Move around from time to time if the position is not comfortable. Maintaining an uncomfortable position may cause back pain. Since this general position is a bit awkward, there is no exact placement for the legs and arms. *Remember to breathe!*

The Sun Star

Fasten your seat belt and get ready for takeoff. I have come up with a group healing technique that I call a Sun Star, and people using this technique have had wonderful and profound experiences. Many have said that the experience has brought them into incredibly quiet states of consciousness, spiritual experiences, or out-of-body experiences. A few people have commented that the changes that take place in their body have felt extremely uncomfortable for the first five or ten minutes, before they started to feel wonderful. Each person in the circle needs to commit to doing this for at least 15 or more minutes.

Have an even number of people arrange themselves in the pattern as illustrated on the previous page. Each person is sending energy through their hands into two other people's feet. You can use group toning, vortexing, chakra spinning, amplified resonance techniques and of course, the fire breath. The more experienced and powerful each member of the group is, the more amazing the results. The synergy of so many different vibrations all mixing together is an incredible and delightful experience. Besides this, the Sun Star is a whole lot of fun.

Holding a Partner

Something as simple as embracing another person, whether standing or laying down can take on new meaning and quality of experience if you are both running the energy through your entire body and out your hands while you embrace. The longer you embrace, the more energy is exchanged.

Remember to breathe!

Sex – How to Make a Good Thing Even Better

Practicing these techniques with a lover can bring a whole new dimension of pleasure to this work. It is a great way to connect, release stress, and become attuned to each other so your vibrations are more compatible. When both people know how to run the energy through their own body and into each other, Quantum-Touch can prolong sensuous pleasure and intensify intimate orgasmic experiences for a more dynamic and exciting sex life. Running energy is also great for foreplay. The key is to practice together. When you do this, you are naturally healing and sharing energy.

Group Hug

Even the ordinary "group hug" can become something quite special if all the people are using Quantum-Touch to run the energy through their hands while the hug is taking place. Remember to keep breathing. This works even better if you have your shoes off and gently pace the front of your foot over the toes of a person standing next to you so that everyone is connected. Try resting your hands on the spine at the bottom of the neck, or in the middle of the lower back.

Work with What You Know

Take any healing technique and combine it with Quantum-Touch. Acupuncturists have told me that it has transformed their practice to run energy into patients after the needles have been inserted. Reflexologists have similarly been impressed when combining Quantum-Touch with reflexology points. Use what you know.

The point of this chapter is to free you up to have fun and experiment with the energy. One friend told me that the other workers in her office have been jealous because when her boss passes out roses to all the workers each month, her rose always lasts so much longer than the others do. Her secret is that she runs energy into the flower and the water. Go ahead and experiment, become playful, and tell me what you have found out.

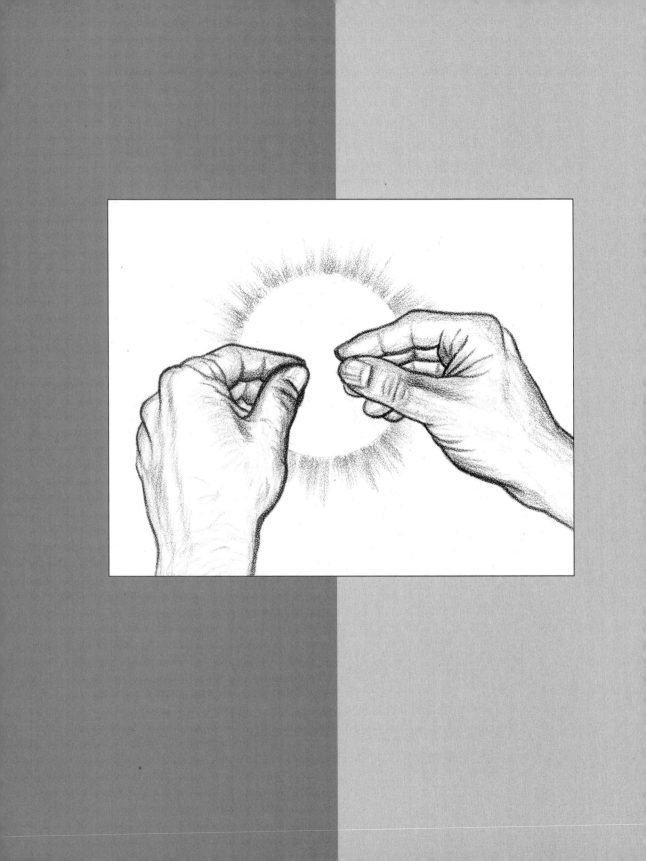

Chapter 15

The Future of Energy Healing

*Energy is the real substance behind
the appearance of matter and forms.*

– Dr. Randolph Stone

Imagine

I believe that this is a good time to share a dream that I have been holding for over twenty years, and in this pivotal time, perhaps this dream can take root and begin to manifest. From a part deep within myself, like a silent prayer, I have been holding a vision close to my heart. I imagine a future where the life-force is universally accepted as being real — real in the same sense that we accept magnetism and gravity. While there is an increasingly popular awareness of ki, chi, and prana, in scientific circles, life-force energy is still considered little more than myth or folklore.

So come join me in my wondering, if you will, and consider what would the world would be like if the consensus was that the life-force was real. Having new tools to measure or evaluate the impact of life-force would be like putting on a new pair of glasses with which to view the world. Every facet of life could be seen in terms of whether it increased the life-force or diminished it – and whole new sets of choices could be made. To give but a few examples:

- When the life-force is considered real, I imagine a new branch of science established that will be called "Life-Force Science," which would be vigorously studied in every prestigious college and university. Discoveries would be made at an extraordinary rate of speed, and the acceptance of the very energy that differentiates that which is alive from that which is dead would finally be acknowledged. The understanding that consciousness affects matter through the function of life-force would have a profound impact on the studies of physics, chemistry, biology, medicine, and psychology.

- When the life-force is considered real, I see healers working in every hospital, every emergency room, and every ambulance. Groups of healers would work on patients a few times a day. Dr.

Norman Shealy suggested that patients in critical care could receive round-the-clock group Quantum-Touch sessions. Healing sessions would routinely be given before, during, and after surgery. By today's standards of patient recovery, the healing would look like something out of science fiction. When the insurance companies figure how many billions of dollars they will save by paying for Quantum-Touch sessions, I believe that we will see this work implemented.

- I envision a day when every child will learn to do healing work in preschool. When a child falls down and hurts herself, the other children will naturally rush in and do healing sessions. When a child is hyperactive and causing problems in class, instead of punishment, the teacher can ask the kids who among them would like to give this child love. By the time each child finishes their education, they would all be amazingly powerful and wonderful healers.

- When the life-force is accepted, I expect to see the day when people are naturally and casually doing healing sessions on each other whenever it is necessary and wherever they are at the time – in line at the movie theater, in a bookstore, at a party, in a train station, anywhere people happen to be.

- When life-force is accepted, I expect that all professional sports teams will travel with a team of accomplished practitioners. There is no question that this work will accelerate the healing of injuries.

- I can imagine life-force healing work being widely used in both developed and third-world countries.

- Finally, I can imagine that there will be breakthroughs with this work that I cannot begin to imagine today.

In these times, scientists seem to be the modern priests who tell the world what is so and what is not so, and I believe that there can be great value working with the double-blind scientific model. Skeptical scientists are quick to point out that this "so-called energy" we like to talk about is not energy at all since it does no "work" on the physical plane. "Work" is a precise term that physicists use to describe how energy affects matter. Numerous experiments by Dr. Bernard Grad at McGill University in Montreal in the 1960s found that among other effects, healers were able to cause a slight but measurable decrease in the surface tension of water. Changing the hydrogen bonding of water and affecting surface tension is clearly a demonstration of "work" on the physical plane.

More recently, Dr. Glen Rein, Ph.D., and director of the Quantum Biology Research Lab in Northport, New York, conducted similar experiments showing that healers were able to cause DNA samples to wind tighter or looser based upon the intentions of the practitioner. I believe it is only a matter of time before we conclusively prove that what we call "energy" truly is energy, even from the point of view of physics.

I believe that it is also necessary to prove that the life-force is not a psychological phenomenon. To test this, we will approach universities and tell them that we have a "placebo therapy" that is getting unreasonably good results, and we would like to understand the "psychological mechanism." A simple test could be designed to work with people who have just had their wisdom teeth extracted. One group would receive a real session with the hands placed lightly over the jaw. A second group would receive an identical session with an untrained practitioner, and a third group would receive no session at all. There are new kinds of drugs that are able to block the part of the brain that allows suggestion, placebo, or habituation to function. Some of the subjects would receive these drugs. I believe that the outcome of these experiments would show that the healing was not due to a psychological mechanism. Then when the question arises about what mechanism could account for the results, we can repeat the work of Dr. Bernard Grad or Dr. Glen Rein and show that there is a physical force involved.

If a phenomenon is not due to a psychological mechanism and is caused by an energy force, we now have an argument to discuss the establishment of a new branch of science. I like to think of this as "Life-

Force Science" since the name is universal and would include a myriad of natural healing modalities.

While this may seem abundantly self-evident and obvious to practitioners of energy work, for political, religious, social, and economic reasons, these understandings remain a mystery to the culture at large. I can only imagine how wonderful it would feel to live in a world where the life-force was not only acknowledged, but embraced and cherished.

When life-force is considered real, we will have a new lens through which to view the world. The way we grow food and what we eat will be evaluated in terms of how it affects our life-force. Education will be evaluated by how creative and loving processes enhance the child's life-force. Medical practices can be evaluated by how well the treatments enhance the patient's life-force. The value of exercise, yoga, pranayama, tai chi, and other various kinds of bodywork can take on a new importance. We can see how laughter, the honest expression of emotions, and the impact of love, care, tenderness, and touch enhance the life-force. When we consider the life-force real, we will live in a world that can transform its priorities and be a healthier and more fulfilling place for us all.

I see a day when healing becomes a universal skill, and the level of pain and suffering on the planet is reduced to a small fraction of what we see today. I have seen families drawn close through their practice of healing each other. I foresee a day when the family of humankind can draw closer through the innate and universal power of loving each other with the use of this healing energy.

Biography

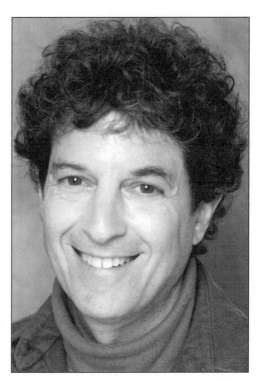

Richard Gordon is recognized as one of the pioneers in the field of energy healing. His book, *Your Healing Hands — The Polarity Experience,* is a best seller that has been translated into nine languages and is a classic guide to energy work. Today, as the founder of Quantum-Touch, Richard is an internationally acclaimed speaker at conferences, medical centers, chiropractic colleges, and holistic health institutes. Mr. Gordon has been on faculty at Heartwood Institute and The Holistic Health Institute.

For information on Quantum-Touch workshops, events, practitioner certification, and other products, contact us at:

Quantum-Touch
P.O. Box 852
Santa Cruz, CA 95061-0852

www.quantumtouch.com

Notes

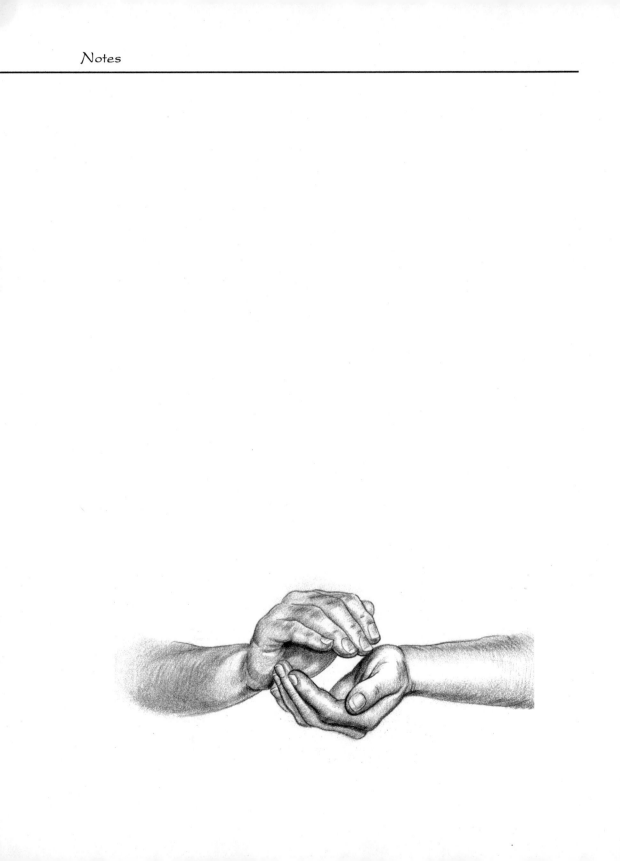